KEY QUESTIONS IN
PAEDIATRICS

Also of interest:

Key Topics in Paediatrics
A.E.M. Davies and A.L. Billson
Publication date July 1994

ISBN 1 872748 58 9

This book describes important issues in child health, and identification and management of problems. The information is presented in a systematic format and provides a concise reference source for all paediatricians and an ideal revision aid for medical students and nursing staff.

KEY QUESTIONS IN
PAEDIATRICS

A.L. Billson
BA MBBS MRCP (UK)
*Senior Registrar in Paediatrics,
Royal United Hospital,
Bath, UK*

A.E.M. Davies
MB ChB MRCP (UK)
*Senior Registrar in Child Health,
Chelsea and Westminster Hospital,
London, UK*

F.O. Finlay
MBBS DCH MRCP (UK)
*Consultant Paediatrician,
Bath and West Community NHS Trust,
Newbridge Hill, Bath, UK*

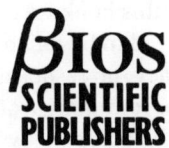

©BIOS Scientific Publishers Limited 1997

First published 1997

All rights reserved. No part of this book may be reproduced or transmitted, in any form or by any means, without permission.

A CIP catalogue record for this book is available from the British Library.

ISBN 1 85996 116 9

BIOS Scientific Publishers Limited,
9 Newtec Place, Magdalen Road, Oxford OX4 1RE, UK.
Tel: +44 (0)1865 726286, Fax: +44 (0)1865 246823.
World Wide Web home page: http://www.Bookshop.co.uk/BIOS/

DISTRIBUTORS

Australia and New Zealand
    DA Information Services
    648 Whitehorse Road, Mitcham
    Victoria 3132, Australia

Singapore and South East Asia
    Toppan Company (S) PTE Ltd
    38 Liu Fang Road, Jurong
    Singapore 2262

India
    Viva Books Private Ltd
    4325/3 Ansari Road, Daryaganj
    New Dehli 110002

USA and Canada
    BIOS Scientific Publishers
    PO Box 605
    Herndon VA 22070

Typeset by Els Boonen, BIOS Scientific Publishers Ltd, Oxford, UK.
Printed by Redwood Books, Trowbridge, UK.

The information contained within this book was obtained by BIOS Scientific Publishers Ltd from sources believed to be reliable. However, while every effort has been made to ensure its accuracy, no responsibility for loss or injury occasioned to any person acting or refraining from action as a result of information contained herein can be accepted by the publishers or authors.

CONTENTS

Abbreviations	vii
Preface	ix

PRACTICE PAPERS

Paper one	1
Paper two	15
Paper three	29
Paper four	43
Paper five	57
Paper six – data interpretation and grey case questions	71

ANSWERS TO PRACTICE PAPERS

Paper one	79
Paper two	87
Paper three	95
Paper four	103
Paper five	111
Paper six	119

ABBREVIATIONS

ACTH	adrenocorticotrophic hormone
AFP	α-feto protein
ALL	acute lymphoblastic leukaemia
AST	aspartate aminotransferase
AV	atrioventricular
Bic	bicarbonate
BP	blood pressure
bpm	beats per minute
CF	cystic fibrosis
CNS	central nervous system
CPK	creatinine phosphokinase
Cr	creatinine
CSF	cerebrospinal fluid
CT	computerized tomography
CXR	chest X-ray
DDAVP	1-D-amino-8-D-arginine vasopression
DKA	diabetic ketoacidosis
DMSA	dimercaptosuccinic acid
ECG	electrocardiogram
EEG	electroencephalogram
ESR	erythrocyte sedimentation rate
FHF	fulminant hepatic failure
FSH	follicle-stimulating hormone
GH	growth hormone
Glu	glucose
GMN	glomerulonephritis
GOR	gastro-oesophageal reflux
Hb	haemoglobin
HBeAg	hepatitis B e-antigen
HBV	hepatitis B virus
HIV	human immunodeficiency virus
HSP	Henoch-Schönlein purpura
HUS	haemolytic uraemic syndrome
ICP	intracranial pressure
IgA	immunoglobulin A
IGF-1	insulin-like growth factor 1
IgM	immunoglobulin M

ITP	idiopathic thrombocytopaenic purpura
i.v.	intravenous
IVH	intraventricular haemorrhage
K	potassium
LH	luteinizing hormone
LIP	lymphocytic interstitial pneumonitis
LP	lumbar puncture
MCV	mean cell volume
MMR	measles, mumps, rubella
Na	sodium
NBT	nitro blue tetrazolium
NEC	necrotizing enterocolitis
NF	neurofibromatosis
NF1	type 1 neurofibromatosis
NF2	type 2 neurofibromatosis
NHL	non-Hodgkin's lymphoma
ORS	oral rehydration solution
OTC	ornithine transcarbamylase
Plt	platelet count
PTH	parathyroid hormone
RDS	respiratory distress syndrome
RTA	renal tubular acidosis
SVT	supraventricular tachycardia
TGA	transposition of the great arteries
TPN	total parenteral nutrition
TSH	thyroid stimulating hormone
U	urea
US	ultrasound
UTI	urinary tract infection
VF	ventricular fibrillation
VLCFA	very long chain fatty acids
VSD	ventricular septal defect
VUR	vesicoureteric reflux
Wbc	white cell count

PREFACE

This book contains 300 multiple choice questions arranged as five practice papers of 60 questions based on the format used for the Diploma in Child Health (DCH) examination. A sixth paper comprises 25 data interpretation and case history questions of the type seen in the current Membership of the Royal College of Physicians (MRCP) Part II (Paediatrics) examination.

The MCQ papers will provide candidates for the DCH with exam practice and enable candidates for the MRCP examination to test their knowledge of the core areas. The reader is encouraged to approach the papers in exam-like conditions and attempt to answer each one within the 2 hours allowed. Medicine is not an exact science with clear cut right or wrong answers to every problem. If you search hard enough you will find an exception to almost every rule. This should not be the approach to multiple choice questions. The examiners are not trying to trick you and efforts are made to ensure that questions are not ambiguous.

The current written examination of MRCP Part II (Paediatrics) includes three sections - case histories (6 questions - time allowed 55 minutes), data interpretation (10 questions - time allowed 45 minutes), and slide interpretation (20 slides). For many MRCP candidates the data interpretation section is the most difficult part of the examination. In this book, paper six consists of 25 mixed data interpretation and case history questions which will be useful for revision purposes. Many of the topics covered appear regularly in this part of the exam. It is hoped that these questions will prompt thought and discussion, leading to a better understanding of the subjects.

Answers to all the questions are provided at the back of the book with brief explanations where needed. The reader is referred to the appropriate topic in Key Topics in Paediatrics for a background to the questions and its answers.

Finally, if you feel that the answer given to any particular question in this book is incorrect, please do not hesitate to let us know.

Amanda Billson
Anne Davies
Fiona Finlay

PRACTICE PAPER ONE

Allow 2 hours for the completion of all 60 questions
Answers are on page 79

1.1 **Oliguria secondary to hypovolaemia**

A should be treated with diuretics
B is associated with a low urinary sodium concentration
C may occur in nephrotic syndrome
D occurs in tumour lysis syndrome
E is usually reversible with volume expansion

1.2 **Congenital adrenal hyperplasia is**

A an X-linked recessive disorder
B most commonly due to 17-hydroxyprogesterone deficiency
C a cause of precocious puberty
D due to an enzyme deficiency in the biosynthetic pathway of cortisol from cholesterol
E the most common cause of ambiguous genitalia

1.3 **Iron deficiency anaemia is associated with**

A prematurity
B introduction of solids at 14–16 weeks of age
C continued use of formula milk after 9 months of age
D β–thalassaemia trait
E a high intake of dietary phytates

1.4 **In supraventricular tachycardia (SVT)**

A there is usually an underlying structural heart defect
B 30–40% of cases present in the first few weeks of life
C the heart rate is usually between 150 and 200 bpm
D DC cardioversion is the treatment of choice if the child is cardiovascularly stable
E adenosine acts by slowing conduction from the sino-atrial node

1.5 Secretion of parathyroid hormone

    A is higher in the morning than the evening
    B is increased by hypercalcaemia
    C increases renal hydroxylation of 25-hydroxy vitamin D
    D decreases renal excretion of phosphate
    E is increased in vitamin D deficient rickets

1.6 When providing basic life support to an infant

    A the neck should be flexed to clear the airway
    B the correct site for cardiac compression is one finger breadth below the xiphisternum
    C palpation of the carotid artery is the easiest site for detection of a central pulse
    D cardiac compressions should be commenced if the pulse rate is 50 bpm
    E a ratio of five cardiac compressions to one breath should be maintained

1.7 Complications of chronic renal failure include

    A megaloblastic anaemia
    B bone pain
    C type 1 hyperlipidaemia
    D anorexia
    E polyuria

1.8 Metabolic disturbances which can directly cause acute encephalopathy include

    A hypoglycaemia
    B hyperglycaemia
    C hyponatraemia
    D hypokalaemia
    E hypercalcaemia

1.9   Congenital heart disease is

       A cyanotic in 70% of cases
       B associated with a non-cardiac anomaly in 10–15% of affected children
       C found in <25% of children with Down's syndrome
       D associated with maternal pre-eclampsia
       E three times more common if there is a previously affected sibling

1.10   Characteristic features of Down's syndrome include

       A flat occiput
       B clinodactyly
       C increased risk of Hirschsprung's disease
       D sensorineural deafness
       E early cataracts

1.11   Childhood diabetes mellitus

       A should only be diagnosed after performing a glucose tolerance test
       B is more common in sub-Saharan Africa than in northern Europe
       C is associated with an increased incidence of Hashimoto's thyroiditis
       D has a prevalence of 1 in 1200 school children in the UK
       E usually presents with ketoacidosis

1.12   Enuresis

       A has an underlying organic cause in approximately 15% of cases
       B occurs in approximately 5% of children aged 10 years
       C should be treated with drug therapy if it persists beyond the age of 5 years
       D is often familial
       E resolves by the age of 15 years in all cases

1.13   In glomerulonephritis (GMN)

       A the urine is usually frothy
       B there may be a family history of sensorineural deafness
       C a rise in complement levels (C3 and C4) is usually seen
       D renal biopsy is essential
       E acute hypertensive encephalopathy is common

1.14 Growth hormone (GH) insufficiency is

    A reliably diagnosed by a clonidine stimulation test
    B often seen in children who have received high-dose cranial irradiation
    C the most likely diagnosis if a child's growth velocity is less than 4 cm/year
    D treated with intravenous infusions of biosynthetic GH
    E associated with high levels of insulin-like growth factor 1 (IGF-1)

1.15 There is an increased risk of renal tract calculi formation in a child with

    A a neuropathic bladder
    B cystinosis
    C distal renal tubular acidosis
    D idiopathic hypercalciuria
    E hypothyroidism

1.16 The following statements are correct about laws relating to children

    A an emergency protection order lasts for 24 hours
    B a child assessment order is used in cases of immediate physical risk
    C a care order places the parental responsibility with social services
    D children should give their own consent to medical treatment if they have sufficient understanding
    E a contact order determines who the child should live with

1.17 Haemophilia B (Christmas disease)

    A tends to have more severe clinical manifestations than haemophilia A
    B is treated with regular infusions of cryoprecipitate
    C may lead to joint deformity and ankylosis
    D is asymptomatic in carriers
    E is an autosomal recessive condition

1.18 Clinical features of heart failure in infancy include

    A hepatomegaly
    B bradycardia
    C improvement in symptoms over the first 6 weeks of life
    D sweating
    E poor feeding

1.19 **Cleft lip**

   A is more common in girls
   B occurs in Patau's syndrome
   C is more common on the right
   D most commonly shows polygenic inheritance
   E may be associated with renal tract abnormalities

1.20 **Central nervous system involvement in leukaemia is**

   A common at diagnosis
   B best diagnosed by CT scan
   C sometimes asymptomatic
   D a poor prognostic indicator
   E an indication for cranial irradiation

1.21 **A 9-month-old girl should be able to**

   A build a tower of 3–4 bricks
   B sit unsupported
   C transfer objects from hand to hand
   D walk upstairs with hand held
   E demonstrate a pincer grip

1.22 **Neonatal respiratory distress syndrome (RDS) is**

   A seen in most babies of birth weight <2.5 kg
   B more common in infants of diabetic mothers
   C associated with prolonged rupture of the membranes
   D less severe in babies of Afro-Caribbean origin than Caucasians
   E exacerbated by hypothermia

1.23 **Factors predisposing a baby to develop necrotizing enterocolitis (NEC) include**

   A breast feeding
   B hypotension
   C birth weight <1500 g
   D patent ductus arteriosus
   E intra-uterine growth retardation

1.24 In nephrotic syndrome

A abdominal pain may be a symptom of hypovolaemia
B hyperlipidaemia is common
C renal biopsy is usually indicated
D there is an increased bleeding tendency
E treatment with cyclophosphamide should be considered if relapse occurs within 1 year

1.25 Urine osmolality

A should fall during water deprivation
B rises with the administration of DDAVP in nephrogenic diabetes insipidus
C is appropriately low in psychogenic polydipsia
D is rarely over 200 mosmol/l in central diabetes insipidus
E is low in early pre-renal failure

1.26 Factors predisposing to preterm delivery include

A twin pregnancy
B Afro-Caribbean origin
C smoking
D social class 1
E previous preterm delivery

1.27 In normal pubertal development

A 95% of girls will have commenced puberty before the age of 14 years
B luteinizing hormone stimulates spermatogenesis in boys
C luteinizing hormone stimulates ovulation in girls
D increase in testicular volume to 4 ml is the first sign of puberty in boys
E the growth spurt occurs earlier in girls than boys

1.28 In Henoch–Schönlein purpura (HSP)

A joint swelling almost always occurs before the appearance of the purpuric rash
B microscopic haematuria occurs in about 10% of cases
C the prothrombin time is prolonged
D symptoms usually resolve within 2–6 weeks
E intussusception is a recognized complication

1.29 Features of chronic lead poisoning include

   A constipation
   B macrocytic anaemia
   C basophilic stippling
   D behavioural problems
   E low plasma concentration of δ-aminolaevulinic acid

1.30 Infants of diabetic mothers are at increased risk of

   A shoulder dystocia
   B jaundice
   C respiratory distress syndrome
   D sacral agenesis
   E hypertrophic cardiomyopathy

1.31 Factors predisposing to intracranial venous occlusion include

   A protein C deficiency
   B sinusitis
   C moya-moya disease
   D polycythaemia
   E polyarteritis nodosa

1.32 Whooping cough

   A occurs in epidemics at 10-yearly intervals in the UK
   B has an incubation period of 7–10 days
   C typically causes a neutrophil leucocytosis
   D is known as the 100 day cough
   E is no longer included in the UK immunization schedule

1.33 With regard to allergic reactions

   A type 1 is cell-mediated hypersensitivity
   B type 3 is the Arthus phenomenon
   C type 4 is a cytotoxic reaction
   D type 2 is an immediate hypersensitivity reaction
   E type 3 is immune complex mediated

1.34 Features of autism include

   A abnormal expressive language
   B avoidance of gaze
   C difficulty separating from parents
   D lack of symbolic play
   E ritualistic behaviours

1.35 In a cyanosed baby

   A an arterial pO_2 of > 14 kPa in 80–100% oxygen excludes a major left-to-right shunt
   B the lung fields may be plethoric on chest X-ray
   C a superior axis on ECG is suggestive of transposition of the great arteries
   D right-to-left shunting through the ductus arteriosus and foramen ovale may persist following intrapartum asphyxia
   E indomethacin is used to maintain blood flow through the ductus arteriosus

1.36 Following a near-drowning episode a child may develop

   A reduced intracranial pressure
   B gross electrolyte imbalance
   C hyperthermia
   D cardiac arrhythmias
   E respiratory distress

1.37 Known teratogens include

   A sodium valproate
   B toxoplasmosis
   C folic acid
   D organic solvents
   E warfarin

1.38 Amino acid disorders include

   A phenylketonuria
   B maple syrup urine disease
   C citrullinaemia
   D tyrosinaemia
   E galactosaemia

1.39 Major features of rheumatic fever include

   A subcutaneous nodules
   B chorea
   C prolonged PR interval on ECG
   D erythema marginatum
   E raised ESR

1.40 Indications for adenotonsillectomy include

   A obstructive sleep apnoea
   B ciliary dyskinesia
   C peritonsillar abscess
   D recurrent sinusitis
   E investigation of malignancy

1.41 In coeliac disease

   A the presenting feature may be microcytic anaemia
   B the presence of circulating antigliadin antibodies is diagnostic
   C there is an increased risk of carcinoma of the oesophagus in adulthood
   D barium meal and follow-through is a useful investigation in suspected cases
   E the presence of a flat jejunal mucosa on biopsy is diagnostic

1.42 In a child presenting with acute abdominal pain

   A the cause may be a primary infection with *Streptococcus pneumoniae*
   B Crohn's disease is a common cause
   C pus cells in the urine indicate a urinary tract infection
   D right iliac fossa pain may be caused by torsion of the testis
   E Gram-negative antibiotic cover should be given if mesenteric nodes are found to be enlarged at laparotomy

1.43 Recognized features of Sturge–Weber syndrome are

   A a port-wine stain over the ophthalmic division of the trigeminal nerve
   B leptomeningeal angiomatosis in all cases
   C glaucoma
   D 'rail-road' track calcification on skull X-ray from birth
   E hemiplegia

1.44 Atopic eczema

A affects 3% of pre-school children
B causes intense itching as the predominant symptom
C often affects the perineum
D causes poor sleep patterns
E is a cause of short stature

1.45 Kawasaki disease

A is a tick-borne disease
B affects predominantly pre-school children
C is more common in Oriental races than Caucasians
D has a prevalence in the UK of approximately 3 per 1000
E has a seasonal variation in incidence

1.46 In acute laryngotracheobronchitis (croup)

A parainfluenza virus is a common causative agent
B a 'barking' cough is a prominent feature
C the child is usually of school age
D restlessness indicates good respiratory effort
E nebulized adrenaline may give temporary relief

1.47 Selective IgA deficiency is

A relatively common, affecting 1 in 500 in the Caucasian populations
B often asymptomatic
C usually the underlying cause in a child with recurrent meningococcal disease
D associated with autoimmune disorders
E a cause of recurrent pulmonary infection

1.48 Causes of generalized lymphadenopathy include

A Gaucher's disease
B carbamazepine therapy
C chronic granulomatous disease
D aplastic anaemia
E Epstein–Barr virus infection

1.49 Features of fulminant hepatic failure (FHF) include

   A hypoglycaemia
   B truncal rash
   C vomiting
   D aggressive behaviour
   E tachypnoea

1.50 Infection with Listeria monocytogenes

   A should be considered if Gram-negative rods are seen in the CSF
   B may cause meningitis in the neonatal period
   C is a cause of intra-uterine growth retardation
   D usually responds to ampicillin and gentamicin
   E occurs in outbreaks associated with ingestion of soft cheese

1.51 Gastro-oesophageal reflux (GOR)

   A occurs physiologically
   B may cause respiratory symptoms
   C is most reliably diagnosed by barium meal
   D may be treated with cisapride
   E may present with iron deficiency anaemia

1.52 The risk of vertical transmission of HIV infection is

   A ~15% in untreated women in the UK
   B increased by breast feeding
   C increased if the mother is infected during the pregnancy
   D reduced by Caesarean section
   E increased if there is premature delivery

1.53 In the management of acute gastroenteritis

   A breast feeding should be discontinued for 24 hours
   B oral rehydration solution (ORS) is effective in the rehydration of most moderately dehydrated patients
   C proprietary oral rehydration solutions in the UK contain 35–60 mmol/l of sodium
   D antidiarrhoeal agents are indicated if stool losses are severe
   E acidosis during severe dehydration should be corrected with i.v. sodium bicarbonate

1.54 Total parenteral nutrition (TPN)

A should only be introduced during a period of complete bowel rest
B may be given via a peripheral vein
C may be complicated by cholestatic jaundice
D is contra-indicated in the presence of thrombocytopenia
E is indicated in chronic intestinal pseudo-obstruction

1.55 Conditions with X-linked recessive inheritance include

A haemophilia
B Duchenne's muscular dystrophy
C colour blindness
D ornithine transcarbamylase (OTC) deficiency
E chronic granulomatous disease

1.56 Cerebral palsy

A is a progressive disorder of movement and posture
B is associated with an increased incidence of hip dislocation
C has an estimated prevalence of 0.4 per 1000 live births
D has a clear aetiological factor in approximately 60% of cases
E is commonly dyskinetic when due to neonatal hyperbilirubinaemia

1.57 Causes of skin blistering include

A insect bites
B Epstein–Barr virus
C eczema
D erythema multiforme
E Coxsackie A16 virus

1.58 Features of chronic non-specific (toddler) diarrhoea are

A nocturnal diarrhoea
B food particles and mucus in the stool
C normal growth velocity
D alternating constipation and diarrhoea
E increased incidence of urinary tract infection

1.59 **A simple febrile convulsion**

    A will occur in 0.5–1% of children between the ages of 6 months and 6 years
    B may leave a residual Todd's paresis
    C will recur in 30% of affected children
    D lasts less than 15 minutes
    E is associated with a very low risk of later epilepsy in a child with no pre-existing neurodevelopmental abnormality

1.60 **Guttate psoriasis**

    A is often preceded by streptococcal tonsillitis
    B may resolve spontaneously
    C occurs along sites of skin injury (Koebner phenomenon)
    D particularly affects knees and elbows
    E typically causes nail changes

PRACTICE PAPER TWO

Allow 2 hours for the completion of all 60 questions
Answers are on page 87

2.1   **In acute renal failure**

    A oliguria is defined as a urine output of <200 ml/m^2/day
    B a raised urine osmolality:plasma osmolality ratio excludes a pre-renal cause
    C hypertension is secondary to salt and water overload
    D calcium resonium is given i.v. to reduce the cardiotoxic effects of hyperkalaemia
    E hypernatraemia is common

2.2   **Glucocorticoid excess**

    A is usually due to increased endogenous glucocorticoid production
    B in Cushing's syndrome is due to an ACTH-secreting pituitary adenoma
    C predisposes to aseptic necrosis of the hip
    D causes muscle weakness
    E antagonizes insulin

2.3   **In hereditary spherocytosis**

    A the inheritance is X-linked recessive
    B the direct Coombs' test is usually positive
    C regular blood transfusions are required
    D haemolysis may be precipitated by ingestion of fava beans
    E splenectomy is the treatment of choice in the first decade

2.4   **In heart block**

    A the PR interval is usually >0.20 sec
    B complete AV dissociation is known as the Wenckebach phenomenon
    C digitalis toxicity may be the cause
    D the child may be asymptomatic
    E maternal lupus should be suspected if presentation is in the neonatal period

2.5 Defective bone mineralization results from

    A renal phosphate loss in vitamin D-resistant rickets
    B primary hyperparathyroidism in chronic renal failure
    C inadequate calcium intake in premature infants
    D dietary vitamin D deficiency in the majority of cases
    E reduced gastrointestinal absorption of calcium in Fanconi syndrome

2.6 A child in asystole

    A should be given adrenaline 10 µg/kg i.v. as the first drug
    B has a very good prognosis if resuscitated successfully
    C should be ventilated with a high concentration of oxygen if the initial resuscitation with two doses of adrenaline is not successful
    D is treated with a DC shock of 2 J/kg
    E may be hypovolaemic

2.7 Indications for renal dialysis include

    A fluid overload
    B worsening hyperkalaemia
    C asymptomatic uraemia
    D worsening acidosis
    E renal osteodystrophy

2.8 In a child presenting with an acute encephalopathy

    A flexion of the arms and extension of the legs is a decerebrate posture
    B a fixed dilated pupil suggests ipsilateral tentorial herniation of the brain
    C the cerebral perfusion pressure is equal to the mean arterial blood pressure minus the intracranial pressure
    D the Glasgow coma score should be assessed before any other intervention
    E absence of papilloedema excludes raised intracranial pressure

2.9 In a child with a ventricular septal defect

    A the murmur is typically soft and varies with the position of the child
    B the ECG may be normal
    C there is a right-to-left shunt
    D surgical closure is usually required
    E prophylactic antibiotics should be given when undergoing dental extractions

2.10 **A seven-week-old baby boy**

   A lies prone with a flat pelvis
   B turns towards sound
   C smiles in response to his mother
   D follows objects from the side to the midline
   E holds an object if it is placed in his hand

2.11 **In an insulin dependent diabetic**

   A the insulin dose should be reduced if the child is not eating during an intercurrent upper respiratory tract infection
   B monitoring of glycaemic control is best done by urinalysis
   C glycosylated haemoglobin levels give an index of glycaemic control over the previous 2–3 months
   D increased insulin requirements during puberty are due to poor diet
   E a low fat, high fibre diet should be encouraged

2.12 **In a child with secondary enuresis**

   A an ectopic ureter opening into the urethra is likely
   B urinalysis may be helpful
   C renal tract ultrasound is indicated
   D constipation should be excluded
   E reward systems such as star charts are rarely helpful

2.13 **Post-streptococcal glomerulonephritis**

   A usually causes mild renal impairment
   B is a recognized cause of acute hypertensive encephalopathy
   C has a poor prognosis if microscopic haematuria persists for >6 months
   D is usually managed with short-term peritoneal dialysis
   E is an immune complex disorder

2.14 **Growth velocity**

   A remains remarkably constant over a 12-month period
   B decreases during childhood
   C reaches a peak of 7–12 cm/year during puberty
   D below the 25th centile for 2 consecutive years requires investigation
   E is usually low for pubertal stage in constitutional short stature

2.15 Microscopic haematuria is

A usually intermittent in IgA nephropathy
B a common presenting symptom of Wilms' tumour
C most commonly due to primary glomerular disease in childhood
D uncommon in Henoch–Schönlein purpura
E associated with hypertension and oliguria in post-streptococcal glomerulonephritis

2.16 The following are characteristic of salicylate poisoning

A hypoventilation
B hyperglycaemia
C hypothermia
D dehydration
E tinnitus

2.17 In haemophilia A

A a family history is common
B a factor VIII level 20% of normal is associated with severe bleeding problems
C desmopressin infusions can be used to reduce bleeding during dental extractions
D physiotherapy is contra-indicated after a joint bleed
E factor VIII-related antigen levels are low

2.18 Complications of perinatal asphyxia include

A hyponatraemia
B meconium aspiration
C thrombocytopenia
D hypokalaemia
E patent ductus arteriosus

2.19 Complications of hypertension include

A dyspnoea
B migraine
C facial palsy
D accelerated atherosclerosis
E seizures

2.20 Adverse prognostic features in a child with acute leukaemia include

A age <2 years
B a high white cell count at diagnosis
C T cell ALL
D CNS disease
E relapse during treatment

2.21 Causes of hyperammonaemia include

A galactosaemia
B treatment with asparaginase
C ornithine transcarbamylase (OTC) deficiency
D proteus urinary tract infection
E phenylketonuria

2.22 Complications of neonatal meconium aspiration include

A pneumothorax
B atelectasis
C surfactant deficiency
D bronchopulmonary dysplasia
E secondary bacterial infection

2.23 Oesophageal atresia

A occurs in 1 in 3000 live births
B is associated with oligohydramnios
C is always associated with a tracheo-oesophageal fistula
D may precipitate pre-term delivery
E presents with a scaphoid abdomen

2.24 Nephrotic syndrome

A is a common condition with a prevalence of 6 per 1000 children
B is more common in boys than girls
C is usually steroid resistant in childhood
D usually follows a streptococcal sore throat
E may present at birth

2.25 **Distal renal tubular acidosis (RTA) is**

    A more common than proximal RTA
    B a cause of muscle weakness
    C associated with increased bicarbonate loss from the renal tubules
    D a cause of hyperkalaemic acidosis
    E associated with nephrocalcinosis

2.26 **In a premature infant**

    A the chance of survival at 28 weeks gestation is <25%
    B retinopathy of prematurity is more common if the birth weight is <1000 g
    C with post-haemorrhagic hydrocephalus, ventricular dilatation often becomes static or resolves
    D who has suffered intra-uterine growth retardation, there is an increased risk of necrotizing enterocolitis
    E hypothermia can exacerbate respiratory distress

2.27 **Precocious puberty is**

    A more common in girls
    B usually idiopathic in boys
    C associated with a delayed bone age
    D an indication for CNS imaging in boys
    E more common in children with hydrocephalus

2.28 **Neuroblastoma**

    A has a very poor prognosis in infants under 1 year
    B may present with non-specific malaise
    C is a recognized cause of flaccid paralysis of the lower limbs
    D usually presents with disease localized to the adrenal glands
    E is routinely screened for in the UK during infancy

2.29 **Acquired hypothyroidism is**

    A usually due to autoimmune thyroiditis in the UK
    B more common in girls than boys
    C more common in girls with Turner's syndrome
    D associated with advanced skeletal maturity
    E associated with isolated breast development

2.30 Vesicoureteric reflux (VUR)

 A usually resolves with age
 B is more common in siblings of an affected child
 C is reliably diagnosed by a dimercaptosuccinic acid (DMSA) isotope scan
 D usually requires reimplantation of the ureters
 E is more common in the presence of other renal tract abnormalities

2.31 There is an increased risk of intracranial haemorrhage in

 A antithrombin III deficiency
 B Henoch–Schönlein purpura
 C subacute bacterial endocarditis
 D polycystic disease of the kidneys
 E idiopathic thrombocytopenic purpura

2.32 Features which suggest that a 10-year-old child with acute asthma is having a severe attack include

 A an inability to speak in complete sentences
 B a respiratory rate of 15 breaths/min
 C bilateral wheeze
 D a normal arterial pCO_2
 E confusion

2.33 Complications of infection with *Bordetella pertussis* include

 A subconjunctival haemorrhage
 B pulmonary atelectasis
 C seizures
 D apnoea
 E epistaxis

2.34 The following are features of anaphylaxis

 A vomiting
 B bronchospasm
 C hypertension
 D itching of the mouth
 E stridor

2.35 Non-accidental injury should be considered in the following fractures

    A spiral fractures of long bones
    B fractures of different ages
    C rib fractures
    D epiphyseal fractures of long bones
    E wide skull fractures

2.36 Characteristic features of Edward's syndrome (trisomy 18) include

    A exomphalos
    B micrognathia
    C Brushfield spots
    D an increased risk of leukaemia
    E renal tract abnormalities

2.37 Congenital dislocation of the hip

    A is treated with an adduction splint
    B is more common in girls
    C is associated with a deep acetabulum
    D is best investigated by X-ray in the neonatal period
    E gives rise to a positive Trendelenberg gait as a late sign

2.38 Clinical features of Friedrich's ataxia are

    A dysarthria
    B exaggerated tendon reflexes in the knee and ankle
    C cataracts
    D pes cavus
    E cardiomyopathy

2.39 Rifampicin

    A should be given to kissing contacts of children with meningococcal disease
    B should be given to all household contacts of those with haemophilus meningitis
    C should be given to contacts of children with *streptococcus pneumoniae* meningitis
    D is contra-indicated in pregnancy
    E causes blue–green discolouration of the urine

2.40   In Still's disease

   A   the platelet count is raised
   B   more girls than boys are affected
   C   the rheumatoid factor is positive
   D   antinuclear antibody is negative
   E   onset is usually before the age of 5 years

2.41   The following statements are correct with regard to vision testing

   A   the Snellen chart can be used from 18 months of age
   B   the City University test is used to test colour vision
   C   the Sonksen–Silver test is a test of visual acuity
   D   electroretinography may be useful in neonates
   E   the Ishihara test measures visual acuity

2.42   In a child with Henoch–Schönlein purpura

   A   faecal occult blood indicates the presence of an intussusception
   B   there are characteristic lesions on the lips and mouth
   C   abnormalities of coagulation are common
   D   lesions over the extensor surfaces of the limbs and trunk are typical
   E   increased numbers of megakaryocytes are found in the bone marrow aspirate

2.43   In coeliac disease

   A   symptoms occur during the first 6 months of gluten ingestion
   B   the distal small bowel mucosa is predominantly affected
   C   there is an association with dermatitis herpetiformis
   D   25% of first degree relatives will also have coeliac disease
   E   there is an association with HLA-B8 and -DR3

2.44   In a child suspected of having an intussusception

   A   the typical age at presentation is between 6–12 weeks
   B   a sausage-shaped mass is most commonly felt in the right hypochondrium
   C   the presence of a Meckel's diverticulum may have been a predisposing factor
   D   plain abdominal X-rays are usually unhelpful
   E   a barium meal is a useful initial investigation

2.45 In an infant with Hirschsprung's disease

  A there is incomplete development of myocytes in the longitudinal muscle layer of the large bowel
  B presentation usually occurs during the first week of life
  C there may also be Down's syndrome
  D necrotizing enterocolitis is a feared complication
  E the diagnosis is confirmed by suction rectal biopsy

2.46 In type 1 neurofibromatosis (NF1) (Von Recklinghausen)

  A inheritance is autosomal dominant
  B phaeochromocytoma is a rare complication
  C *cafe au lait* macules usually appear during the first year of life
  D axillary or inguinal freckling is a diagnostic criterion
  E acoustic neuroma is a diagnostic feature

2.47 In the management of atopic eczema

  A paraffin-based creams help with dryness
  B sedatives are contra-indicated
  C streptococcus is a frequent secondary infection
  D secondary skin infection need only be treated with topical antibiotics
  E dietary elimination of dairy products should be tried before topical steroids are commenced

2.48 Diagnostic criteria of Kawasaki disease include

  A cervical lymphadenopathy
  B fever of 5 or more day's duration
  C evidence of recent staphylococcal or streptococcal infection
  D erythema marginatum
  E bilateral conjunctival injection

2.49 In acute epiglottitis

  A *haemophilus influenzae* type B is a causative pathogen
  B a productive cough often precedes the stridor
  C the child prefers to lie down with the neck extended
  D fever is often prominent
  E the stridor is typically loud

2.50 Recognized features of DiGeorge syndrome are

   A hypercalcaemia
   B tetralogy of Fallot
   C eczema
   D defects of humoral immunity
   E facial abnormalities

2.51 Causes of local lymphadenopathy include

   A post vaccination
   B lymphoma
   C phenobarbitone therapy
   D peritonsillar abscess
   E familial hypercholesterolaemia

2.52 Causes of fulminant hepatic failure include

   A paracetamol poisoning
   B hepatitis A virus infection
   C Wilson's disease
   D vitamin D poisoning
   E sodium valproate therapy

2.53 Intra-uterine rubella infection

   A may cause isolated sensorineural deafness
   B can be confirmed by the presence of rubella specific IgM in the first 6 months of life
   C carries the greatest risk to the fetus in the third trimester
   D should be treated with ganciclovir in the neonatal period
   E is a cause of congenital heart disease

2.54 Typical features of hypertrophic pyloric stenosis are

   A preponderance of affected male infants
   B onset of symptoms at birth
   C hypochloraemic alkalosis
   D prolonged jaundice
   E palpable pyloric 'tumour' in the right iliac fossa

2.55 In lymphocytic interstitial pneumonitis (LIP)

　　A　dyspnoea usually precedes chest X-ray changes
　　B　the typical chest X-ray appearance is of bilateral reticulonodular infiltration
　　C　digital clubbing occurs
　　D　clinical improvement with nebulized pentamidine is seen
　　E　haemoptysis is common

2.56 In petit mal epilepsy

　　A　absences are typically induced by breath holding
　　B　the peak age of onset is 6–8 years
　　C　the EEG shows a typical hypsarrhythmia
　　D　response to sodium valproate is usually good
　　E　girls are more commonly affected than boys

2.57 Causes of a reticular rash include

　　A　rubella
　　B　cutaneous polyarteritis nodosa
　　C　human parvovirus B19
　　D　rheumatic fever
　　E　staphylococcal toxic shock syndrome

2.58 Deafness is associated with

　　A　Pendred's syndrome
　　B　Treacher Collins' syndrome
　　C　congenital toxoplasmosis
　　D　Hunter's syndrome
　　E　frusemide therapy in the neonatal period

2.59 Clinical features of rubella infection in childhood include

　　A　occipital lymph gland enlargement
　　B　a pink macular rash lasting 3–4 days
　　C　mucous membrane ulceration
　　D　orchitis
　　E　jaundice

2.60 The diagnosis of cystic fibrosis is

- A possible at 8–10 weeks gestation by chorionic villus sampling in some cases
- B suggested by low levels of immunoreactive trypsin in the neonatal bloodspots
- C excluded if the mutation delta-F508 is absent
- D confirmed by a sweat sodium of 80–120 mmol/l on a sample of 100 mg sweat
- E consistent with a faecal fat excretion of > 5 g/day

PRACTICE PAPER THREE

Allow 2 hours for the completion of all 60 questions
Answers are on page 95

3.1 **Severe hyperkalaemia ($K^+ > 7$ mmol/l) in acute renal failure is**

  A associated with ST depression on ECG
  B lowered by nebulized salbutamol
  C an indication for dialysis
  D usually associated with a metabolic acidosis
  E sometimes seen in haemolytic uraemic syndrome

3.2 **In endocrine disorders**

  A hypertension is a common finding in Bartter's syndrome
  B plasma very long chain fatty acid (VLCFA) concentrations may be raised in adrenal insufficiency
  C hyperaldosteronism results in a hypokalaemic alkalosis
  D insidious onset of lethargy with hyperpigmentation is typical in Conn's syndrome
  E a falling serum potassium may be the first sign of an impending salt-losing crisis in congenital adrenal hyperplasia

3.3 **When using growth charts**

  A only 1 in 250 children will fall below the 0.4th centile on the 1990 nine centile charts
  B the centile lines on a nine centile chart are two-thirds of a standard deviation apart
  C investigation should be considered if a child's height falls across two centile lines within 18–24 months under the age of 5 years
  D the mid-parental height is the sum of the parents heights divided by 2
  E height velocity can be determined from a single height measurement and the bone age

3.4 In cardiology

A a heart rate of <100 bpm in a neonate is always pathological
B atrial fibrillation is the most common arrhythmia in infancy
C a sinus tachycardia is common during a febrile illness
D immersion of a child's face in cold water stimulates the sympathetic nervous system
E supraventricular tachycardia is a recognized cause of hydrops fetalis

3.5 The total serum calcium concentration is

A approximately 40% of the total body calcium
B low in nephrotic syndrome
C increased by parathyroid hormone
D high in stored citrated blood
E high in liver disease

3.6 In the management of paracetamol poisoning

A hepatocellular necrosis is maximal 8–9 days post ingestion
B methionine protects the liver if given within 48 hours of ingestion
C acetylcysteine is given orally
D the prothrombin time should be measured for 3–4 days post ingestion
E acute tubular necrosis may occur

3.7 Chronic renal failure is

A defined as a glomerular filtration rate of <5% of normal
B rarely reversible
C associated with hearing impairment in some children
D almost always secondary to a renal tract malformation
E a cause of polyuria

3.8 Features of Reye's syndrome include

A hypoglycaemia
B hepatomegaly
C seizures
D hyperammonaemia
E raised plasma aspartate aminotransferase (AST)

3.9 Coarcatation of the aorta

- A may present with hypertension alone
- B is found in 10% of girls with Turner's syndrome
- C is excluded if the femoral pulses are present on routine neonatal examination
- D results in right ventricular hypertrophy
- E can be treated by balloon angioplasty

3.10 Contra-indications to immunizations include

- A severe local reaction to a previous dose of the vaccine
- B cough without fever
- C prolonged screaming within 72 hours of a previous dose of the vaccine
- D fever of 38°C within 48 hours of a previous immunization
- E convulsion within 72 hours of a previous immunization

3.11 The following drugs cause ataxia

- A phenytoin
- B digoxin
- C acyclovir
- D piperazine
- E ciprofloxacin

3.12 Sickle cell anaemia

- A is due to a single amino acid substitution in the β-globin chains of haemoglobin
- B usually presents with symptoms in the neonatal period
- C can be diagnosed on cord blood
- D tends to have milder symptoms than the mixed haemoglobinopathy HbS/β-thalassaemia
- E is associated with low fetal haemoglobin concentrations

3.13 Typical features of the acute nephritic syndrome include

- A peak incidence in children aged <5 years
- B preceding streptococcal infection
- C hypoalbuminaemia <25 g/l
- D hypertension
- E oliguria

3.14 **Haemolytic uraemic syndrome (HUS) is associated with**

    A verotoxin producing *E.coli*
    B shigella dysentery
    C crack cocaine
    D a family history of HUS
    E snake bites

3.15 **Chronic bullous dermatosis**

    A predominantly affects teenagers
    B causes blistering in rosette patterns
    C affects the lower half of the body
    D is associated with coeliac disease
    E heals with scarring

3.16 **Congenital hypothyroidism**

    A has an incidence of 1 in 12 000 live births
    B is excluded if the thyroid stimulating hormone (TSH) level is normal on neonatal screening
    C may be transient
    D is associated with an increased risk of learning difficulties if the thyroxine level is <40 nmol/l at diagnosis
    E is associated with delayed bone maturation

3.17 **Urinary tract infection is**

    A a cause of microscopic haematuria
    B more common in girls during the neonatal period
    C most commonly due to *E.coli*
    D associated with failure to thrive in infancy
    E an indication for immediate micturating cystography in all children under 3 years

3.18 **Human parvovirus B19 causes**

    A spontaneous abortion
    B glomerulonephritis
    C arthritis of the small joints
    D erythema infectiosum ('fifth disease')
    E aplastic crises

3.19 Toxic shock syndrome is

　A rapidly progressive
　B a cause of desquamating erythroderma
　C only seen in menstruating girls
　D associated with some viral infections
　E almost invariably associated with thrombocytopenia

3.20 Non-Hodgkin's lymphoma (NHL) is

　A more common in girls
　B usually B cell if arising in the abdomen
　C associated with ataxia telangiectasia
　D most common in adolescents
　E associated with a good prognosis even in advanced disease

3.21 Causes of thrombocytopenia in childhood include

　A neuroblastoma
　B Henoch–Schönlein purpura
　C von Willebrand's disease
　D Gaucher's disease
　E giant haemangiomas

3.22 Recognized causes of facial palsy in childhood include

　A hypertension
　B phenytoin
　C leukaemia
　D Lyme disease
　E salicylate poisoning

3.23 In neonatal surgery

　A gastroschisis is usually associated with other congenital abnormalities
　B diaphragmatic hernia has a better outcome if the defect is repaired within 6 hours of birth
　C necrotizing enterocolitis is usually managed by resection of the affected bowel segment
　D exomphalos is more common than gastroschisis
　E vaginal delivery is contra-indicated if gastroschisis has been diagnosed antenatally

3.24 **Infants who have suffered intra-uterine growth retardation are at increased risk of**

   A polycythaemia
   B necrotizing enterocolitis
   C respiratory distress syndrome
   D thrombocytopenia
   E intrapartum asphyxia

3.25 **In cystinosis**

   A female siblings of an affected boy will not be affected
   B renal tract calculi are common
   C cystine crystals can be identified by slit-lamp examination of the cornea
   D rickets may occur
   E failure to thrive is common

3.26 **Intraventricular haemorrhage (IVH) in a preterm infant**

   A arises directly from the middle cerebral artery
   B occurs in approximately 25% of infants < 1500 g
   C usually occurs during the 3rd or 4th week of life
   D will extend in up to 30% of cases
   E is usually associated with neurological sequelae if limited to the germinal layer

3.27 **Delayed puberty is**

   A a lack of pubertal development in a boy > 15 years or a girl > 14 years
   B usually constitutional
   C associated with McCune Albright's syndrome
   D treated with gonadotrophin releasing hormone analogues
   E an indication for CNS imaging in boys

3.28 **Infantile seborrheic dermatitis**

   A occurs during the first 3 months of life
   B affects both napkin area and scalp
   C causes troublesome itching
   D does not spare skinfolds
   E may be confused with the rash of Langerhan's histiocytosis

3.29 Pain and swelling of joints are features of

   A Henoch–Schönlein purpura
   B rheumatic fever
   C Perthes' disease
   D haemophilia
   E juvenile chronic arthritis

3.30 Central nervous system tumours

   A account for 25% of all childhood malignancy
   B may present with endocrine disturbance
   C commonly metastasize to the liver
   D are nearly always found above the tentorium
   E have an excellent prognosis with surgery alone if completely resected

3.31 Childhood asthma in the UK

   A affects 10–15% of school children
   B causes symptoms by the age of 3 years in 50% of cases
   C is more common if the parents smoke
   D causes the death of 1 in 100 000 children per year
   E subsides spontaneously by puberty in ~75% of cases

3.32 *Mycobacterium tuberculosis* infection in childhood is

   A often asymptomatic
   B non-respiratory in >50% of cases
   C usually diagnosed on sputum culture
   D likely if intradermal tuberculin testing (the Mantoux test) causes a 10 mm wheal
   E no longer a notifiable disease

3.33 Notifiable diseases include

   A mumps
   B dysentery
   C haemolytic uraemic syndrome
   D *Haemophilus influenzae* infection
   E food poisoning

3.34 **Risk factors for child abuse include**

   A poor housing
   B an older mother
   C parental history of abuse as a child
   D last-born child in the family
   E unemployed parents

3.35 **In fragile X syndrome**

   A the fragile site is on the short arm of the X chromosome
   B the testes are small
   C the head circumference is frequently <3rd centile
   D mild learning difficulties are characteristic
   E there is connective tissue dysfunction

3.36 **Causes of global developmental delay include**

   A fragile X syndrome
   B agenesis of the corpus callosum
   C maple syrup urine disease
   D congenital toxoplasmosis
   E cystic hygroma

3.37 **In diabetes mellitus**

   A there is association with HLA-DR3 and -DR4
   B there is an association with mumps
   C there is an increased incidence in spring/summer
   D 80% of affected children have a first degree relative who is diabetic
   E islet cell antibodies are usually detected at diagnosis

3.38 **Irritable hip (transient synovitis)**

   A is associated with an increased erythrocyte sedimentation rate (ESR)
   B is followed by Perthes' disease in 10–15% children
   C resolves after 7–10 days
   D is associated with widening of the joint space on X-ray
   E has a peak age of 2–10 years

3.39 Contra-indications to lumbar puncture in cases of suspected meningitis include

   A unequal pupils
   B petechial rash
   C protracted seizures
   D bulging fontanelle
   E focal neurological signs

3.40 Myasthenia gravis

   A is an autoimmune disorder
   B is more common in boys
   C usually presents with generalized hypotonia
   D is inherited in an autosomal dominant fashion
   E is treated with anticholinesterase inhibitors

3.41 Dermatitis herpetiformis

   A presents as a pruritic vesicular rash on extensor surfaces
   B responds to topical treatment with corticosteroids
   C is associated with asymptomatic gluten-sensitive enteropathy
   D responds to dapsone
   E is an indication for a gluten-free diet

3.42 Acute appendicitis

   A is easiest to diagnose in the pre-school child
   B may present with diarrhoea
   C is typically accompanied by a high swinging fever
   D is frequently associated with a lymphocytosis in the full blood count
   E typically gives a positive faecal occult blood test

3.43 In tuberous sclerosis

   A the typical facial rash (adenoma sebaceum) is due to facial angiofibromata
   B infantile spasms may be the presenting feature
   C cardiac rhabdomyomas may be diagnosed *in utero*
   D renal involvement occurs in 80% of cases
   E intelligence is usually normal

3.44 Clinical features of atopic eczema include

A painless lymphadenopathy
B reticular rash over the cheeks
C white dermographism
D visible extra infra-orbital folds
E the Koebner phenomenon

3.45 In the treatment of Kawasaki disease

A high-dose aspirin should be commenced as soon as possible
B digoxin is contra-indicated
C intravenous acyclovir is indicated if there is mucous membrane involvement
D early use of high-dose immunoglobulin is recommended
E antibiotic prophylaxis for bacterial endocarditis is advised

3.46 Features of chronic granulomatous disease are

A neutrophils which fail to engulf micro-organisms
B osteomyelitis
C staphylococcal skin lesions
D delayed umbilical cord separation
E abnormal nitro blue tetrazolium (NBT) test

3.47 Recognized causes of portal hypertension include

A neonatal umbilical sepsis
B constrictive pericarditis
C homocystinuria
D cystic fibrosis
E congenital hepatic fibrosis

3.48 Toxoplasmosis during pregnancy

A may be asymptomatic in the mother
B is caused by the protozoan *Toxoplasma gondii*
C may cause neonatal hydrocephalus
D is commonly transmitted by the ingestion of undercooked meat
E causes a characteristic macular rash in affected neonates

3.49 **Vomiting**

  A in the early morning is a symptom of an intracranial lesion
  B may be bile stained in an infant with intussusception
  C may be absent in the presence of gastro-oesophageal reflux
  D is a feature of lead poisoning
  E during cytotoxic therapy is effectively prevented by omeprazole

3.50 ***Pneumocystis carinii* pneumonia**

  A prophylaxis in immunosuppressed patients is provided by cotrimoxazole
  B may present with wheezing
  C causes cystic changes on chest X-ray
  D can be diagnosed by bronchoalveolar lavage
  E may present with a fever alone

3.51 **Pathogens responsible for acute gastroenteritis include**

  A *Shigella sonneii*
  B *Campylobacter jejuni*
  C *Giardia lamblia*
  D Coxsackie virus A16
  E *Entamoeba histolytica*

3.52 **Clinical features of infective endocarditis include**

  A finger clubbing
  B splenomegaly
  C Lisch nodules
  D subconjunctival haemorrhages
  E haematuria

3.53 **Features of familial adenomatous polyposis include**

  A massive rectal bleeding
  B autosomal dominant inheritance
  C an association with hepatoblastoma
  D premalignant adenomatous polyps in the colorectum
  E facial angiofibromas

3.54 Features of Gilbert's syndrome are

   A autosomal dominant inheritance
   B positive Coomb's test
   C mild conjugated hyperbilirubinaemia
   D elevation of serum bilirubin on fasting
   E splenomegaly

3.55 Physiological neonatal jaundice

   A does not occur in preterm infants
   B appears during the first 24 hours of life
   C peaks at a bilirubin level of approximately 120 µmol/l in a term infant
   D begins to fade in the third or fourth week of life
   E is associated with decreased red cell survival

3.56 The following conditions cause diarrhoea in the neonatal period

   A necrotizing enterocolitis
   B neonatal hyperthyroidism
   C Hirschsprung's disease
   D congenital microvillous atrophy
   E lactase deficiency

3.57 Gastrointestinal complications of cystic fibrosis include

   A rectal prolapse
   B neonatal meconium ileus
   C malrotation
   D malabsorption
   E recurrent abdominal pain

3.58 Regarding hearing and language development

   A a 5-month-old would be expected to produce two-syllable babble (baba, dada)
   B a 15-month-old would be expected to have at least six words
   C a 2-year-old spontaneously puts together 2–3 word sentences
   D one in 500 children has moderate to severe deafness requiring a hearing aid
   E pure-tone audiometry can be used to test hearing in the neonatal period

3.59 Amniocentesis

- A is performed at 8–12 weeks
- B carries a 1% risk of miscarriage
- C is an indication for anti-D prophylaxis in rhesus negative mothers
- D allows the karyotype of the fetus to be determined within 2–3 days
- E may be indicated if the maternal serum AFP is low

3.60 Typical features of a migraine include

- A a positive family history of migraine in up to 90% of cases
- B unilateral paroxysmal headache
- C headache which is present on morning waking
- D an associated cranial bruit
- E visual disturbance

PRACTICE PAPER FOUR

Allow 2 hours for the completion of all 60 questions
Answers are on page 103

4.1   In a child presenting with diabetic ketoacidosis (DKA)

   A   there is a risk of hyperkalaemia once treatment is commenced
   B   gastric dilatation may occur
   C   intravenous fluids are not necessary if the child weighs 22 kg and is able to drink 45 ml of water/hour
   D   the risk of cerebral oedema is related to the degree of acidosis
   E   the white cell count may be raised even in the absence of infection

4.2   Recognized risk factors for the development of neonatal hypoglycaemia include

   A   intra-uterine growth retardation
   B   perinatal asphyxia
   C   maternal propranolol therapy
   D   rhesus disease
   E   Beckwith–Wiedemann syndrome

4.3   Galactosaemia

   A   is due to galactose-1-phosphate uridyl transferase deficiency
   B   usually presents with prolonged jaundice
   C   gives the infant a peculiar smell
   D   results in a cardiomyopathy
   E   is a cause of glaucoma

4.4   Recognized causes of convulsions in the neonatal period include

   A   hypocalcaemia
   B   maternal opiate abuse
   C   phenylketonuria
   D   hypothyroidism
   E   haemorrhagic disease of the newborn

4.5 Hypocalcaemia due to hypoparathyroidism is associated with

A mucocutaneous candidiasis
B cataracts
C hypophosphataemia
D a rise in urinary cAMP in response to parathyroid hormone
E adrenal insufficiency

4.6 Complications of β-thalassaemia major include

A hypersplenism
B cardiomyopathy
C delayed puberty
D brittle long bones
E liver cirrhosis

4.7 Factors contributing to renal osteodystrophy in chronic renal failure include

A hyperphosphataemia
B hypoparathyroidism
C acidosis
D increased calcium absorption from the gut
E relative vitamin D resistance

4.8 Transient tachypnoea of the newborn

A must settle within the first 4 hours of life to be called transient
B is more common following Caesarean delivery
C can be distinguished from group B streptococcal infection on CXR
D is due to delayed surfactant production
E rarely leads to an oxygen requirement of >40%

4.9 Features of tetralogy of Fallot include

A right ventricular outflow tract obstruction
B left axis deviation on ECG
C ventricular septal defect
D fixed splitting of the second heart sound
E right-to-left shunting

4.10 Cystinuria is

 A a common condition occurring in 1 in 600 of the population
 B associated with renal tract calculi formation in > 75% of affected individuals
 C a cause of rickets
 D diagnosed by slit-lamp examination of the cornea
 E a specific transport defect of dibasic amino acids

4.11 Features of ataxia telangiectasia are

 A autosomal recessive inheritance
 B oculomotor apraxia
 C mental retardation
 D dementia
 E a raised blood α-fetoprotein level

4.12 IgA nephropathy is

 A the most common cause of recurrent painless haematuria in childhood
 B a benign disease
 C due to immune complex deposition on the glomerular basement membrane
 D more common in males than females
 E a cause of persistent microscopic haematuria

4.13 Recognized causes of haemolytic anaemia include

 A mycoplasma infection
 B spherocytosis
 C hookworms
 D phenytoin
 E pyruvate kinase deficiency

4.14 Tall stature is

 A often familial
 B associated with mitral valve prolapse
 C seen at final height in a child with precocious puberty
 D seen in Silver–Russell syndrome
 E usually investigated with pituitary imaging

4.15 Regarding thyroid function

- A thyroid stimulating hormone (TSH) is secreted by the posterior pituitary
- B tri-iodothyronine (T_3) is more metabolically active than thyroxine (T_4)
- C a disorder of thyroid hormone synthesis should be considered if a normal thyroid gland is demonstrated on radioisotope scan in an infant with congenital hypothyroidism
- D treatment of acquired hypothyroidism usually results in an immediate improvement in behaviour
- E hypothyroidism is associated with precocious puberty

4.16 Clinical signs of inadequate tissue perfusion include

- A restlessness
- B grunting respiration
- C capillary refill time <2 sec
- D polyuria
- E tachycardia

4.17 Recognized causes of acute hemiplegia in childhood include

- A herpes simplex infection
- B moya-moya disease
- C migraine
- D protein S deficiency
- E acyanotic congenital heart disease

4.18 Recurrent abdominal pain in childhood is

- A usually organic
- B associated with an increased incidence of irritable bowel symptoms in the parents
- C sometimes responsive to treatment with pizotifen
- D associated with higher intelligence
- E more common in girls

4.19 Symptoms and signs of chronically undertreated asthma include

- A nocturnal cough
- B pectus carinatum
- C short stature
- D clubbing
- E persistent focal crackles or wheezes

4.20 **In the management of a child with a severe scald**

A the volume of fluid (ml) required to replace losses in the first 8 hours after the injury is approximately weight (kg) × % area burned
B transfer to a specialist burns unit is not necessary unless >25% of the body surface area is affected
C inhalational injury should be considered if there are facial burns
D an escharotomy will be needed if the anterior chest wall is affected
E partial thickness scalds heal in 14–21 days in the absence of infection

4.21 **In an infant with acute bronchiolitis**

A the usual pathogen responsible is parainfluenza virus
B recurrent apnoea may initially be the only clinical feature
C recurrent cough and wheeze during the following 12 months is very common
D mechanical ventilation is needed in 20–30% of infants admitted to hospital
E ritodrine is an antiviral agent which may be of benefit if there is an underlying cardiorespiratory disorder

4.22 **Recognized causes of hypertension in childhood include**

A renal artery stenosis
B Bartter's syndrome
C Cushing's syndrome
D Addison's disease
E porphyria

4.23 **Malignancy in childhood**

A is more common in girls
B accounts for less than 5% of all deaths between the ages of 1 and 15 years
C is newly diagnosed in approximately 120 children per year in the UK
D is associated with an increased risk of maternal breast cancer in some families
E is curable in more than 50% of cases overall

4.24 **The following are correct with regard to nerve injuries sustained by an infant during birth**

    A injury of C5, C6 may cause an Erb's palsy
    B facial nerve palsy is usually bilateral
    C Horner's syndrome is due to cervical sympathetic nerve damage
    D damage to C1, C2 causes Klumpke's palsy
    E an arm with a Klumpke's palsy is held in the waiter's tip position

4.25 **In cases of non-accidental injury it must be remembered that**

    A staphylococcal bullous impetigo may be confused with a cigarette burn
    B reflex anal dilatation is a reliable sign of sexual abuse
    C bone fractures may be secondary to copper deficiency
    D gastro-oesophageal reflux may cause apnoeic spells
    E periosteal new bone formation is seen on skeletal survey 4–5 days after a fracture

4.26 **With regard to sleep problems**

    A night terrors occur during rapid eye movement sleep
    B a child will remember sleep walking when he wakes the following morning
    C a child wakes fully during a nightmare with a vivid recollection of the dream
    D night terrors occur in the first third of the night
    E organic illnesses may cause insomnia

4.27 **Turner's syndrome**

    A is associated with normal fertility
    B is characterized by cubitus valgus
    C has a prevalence of 3 per 1000 live births
    D is the only monosomy compatible with life
    E is associated with severe learning difficulties

4.28 The following definitions are correct

   A the infant mortality rate is the number of deaths in the first year of life per 1000 total births
   B the neonatal mortality rate is the number of deaths in the first 27 days of life per 1000 live births
   C the stillbirth rate is the number of infants born after 26 weeks who show no sign of life per 1000 total births
   D the perinatal mortality rate is the number of deaths in the first week per 1000 live births
   E the post-neonatal mortality rate is the number of deaths between 28 days and 1 year of life per 1000 live births

4.29 Developmental regression characteristically occurs in

   A Cornelia de Lange syndrome
   B Batten's disease
   C metachromatic leucodystrophy
   D Sturge–Weber syndrome
   E phenylketonuria

4.30 In poisoning with iron

   A as little as 2 g of elemental iron may be fatal
   B gastric lavage should be avoided
   C desferrioxamine is used to chelate the iron
   D the clinical course classically has four phases of which phase 3 is the quiescent phase
   E cardiovascular collapse, acute encephalopathy and hepatic failure may occur after 16–24 hours

4.31 Features of fetal alcohol syndrome include

   A growth retardation
   B learning difficulties
   C short palpebral fissures
   D a smooth philtrum
   E hydrocephalus

4.32 In the management of enuresis

A radiological investigations are mandatory
B urine culture should be performed
C tricyclic drugs work through antimuscarinic effects
D desmopressin is given intra-muscularly
E the pad and buzzer method is only useful in young children

4.33 In failure to thrive

A a specific organic cause is usually identified
B diagnosis is based on serial measurements over time
C mid-upper arm circumference is a useful indicator of muscle bulk
D the weight is below the 0.4th centile by definition
E neutropenia is associated with Schwachman–Diamond syndrome

4.34 Causes of a 'floppy' infant include

A Prader–Willi syndrome
B glycogen storage disorders
C Ehlers–Danlos
D achondroplasia
E hypercalcaemia

4.35 Clinical features of hydrocephalus in infancy include

A dilated scalp veins
B drowsiness
C restriction of downward gaze
D papilloedema
E large anterior fontanelle

4.36 Pertussis vaccine is

A a live vaccine
B given as a triple vaccine combined with the diphtheria and measles vaccines
C contra-indicated in Down's syndrome
D given at 4, 6 and 8 months of age
E given as a booster prior to school entry

4.37 In septic arthritis

A the small joints are usually affected
B streptococcus is the most common infecting organism
C radiology may reveal widening of the joint space
D optimum duration of treatment is 1 week
E multiple joints are often affected in neonates

4.38 Guillain–Barré syndrome is

A a cause of spastic paralysis
B usually self-limiting
C less likely to recover spontaneously if the paralysis is rapidly progressive
D associated with ataxia in some children
E associated with a raised CSF protein

4.39 Cerebro-spinal fluid

A glucose is low in viral meningitis
B polymorphs are raised in bacterial meningitis
C protein is low in bacterial meningitis
D lymphocytes are raised in tuberculous meningitis
E glucose is normal in tuberculous meningitis

4.40 In dystrophia myotonica

A inheritance is autosomal dominant
B ptosis is a feature
C there is difficulty initiating a hand grasp
D there are severe learning difficulties
E the gene has been identified on chromosome 19

4.41 Bone pain without swelling may be caused by

A osteosarcoma
B osteomyelitis
C leukaemia
D osteoid osteoma
E neuroblastoma

4.42 In polyarticular juvenile chronic arthritis

    A seven or more joints are involved
    B uveitis is common
    C cytotoxic agents are widely used in treatment
    D the major features at onset are systemic
    E gold is a disease modifying drug

4.43 The following are inherited as autosomal dominant conditions

    A neurofibromatosis
    B ataxia telangiectasia
    C myotonic dystrophy
    D incontinentia pigmenti
    E congenital spherocytosis

4.44 The following are true with regard to sinusitis

    A a purulent discharge may be seen
    B surgical drainage is required in ~10% of cases
    C complications include periorbital cellulitis
    D immunodeficiency should be considered if sinusitis is chronic
    E complications include cavernous sinus thrombosis

4.45 In a child with chronic constipation

    A abdominal pain is a common symptom
    B hypocalcaemia may be the underlying cause
    C laxatives should only be given for 2–4 weeks
    D ultra-short segment Hirschsprung's disease is best excluded on barium enema
    E abdominal X-rays are never indicated

4.46 Typical laboratory features of atopic eczema are

    A a raised IgE
    B thrombocytopenia
    C eosinophilia
    D microcytic anaemia
    E positive antigliadin antibodies

4.47 Congenital laryngeal stridor (laryngomalacia)

   A presents within 4 weeks of birth
   B produces an abnormal cry
   C improves when the infant lies supine
   D commonly causes failure to thrive
   E is associated with micrognathia

4.48 Modified cow's milk formula for infant feeding

   A is predominantly casein based
   B should be given in a volume of 250 ml/kg/day in a term neonate
   C should be replaced by door-step cow's milk at 6 months of age
   D contains approximately 67 kcal per 100 ml
   E is preferable to breast feeding if the mother is iron deficient

4.49 A 2-year-old boy would be expected to

   A walk up and down stairs alone
   B undo buttons
   C build a tower of six bricks
   D draw a man
   E play make believe games

4.50 Problems associated with a cleft lip and palate include

   A glue ear
   B dental malalignment
   C eczema
   D speech delay
   E difficulties with maternal bonding

4.51 Sebaceous naevi

   A commonly occur on the scalp
   B are associated with CNS developmental defects
   C carry a risk of malignant change
   D appear as smooth waxy plaques
   E contain haemangiomatous elements

4.52 Causes of unresolved fever include

　　A diabetes insipidus
　　B neuroblastoma
　　C coeliac disease
　　D familial dysautonomia (Riley–Day syndrome)
　　E liver abscess

4.53 Common respiratory pathogens in cystic fibrosis (CF) are

　　A *Staphylococcus aureus*
　　B *Aspergillus fumigatus*
　　C *Pseudomonas aeruginosa*
　　D *Pseudomonas cepacia*
　　E *Pneumocystis carinii*

4.54 Rectal bleeding in the newborn may be caused by

　　A necrotizing enterocolitis
　　B haemorrhagic disease of the newborn
　　C mid-gut volvulus
　　D cow's milk protein intolerance
　　E salmonella gastroenteritis

4.55 In hepatitis B virus (HBV) infection

　　A viral replication is by reverse transcription
　　B IgM anticore is the first antibody to appear
　　C the risk of vertical transmission is highest if the mother is HBeAg postive
　　D chronic infection is more common in the immuno-compromised host
　　E there is an increased risk of subsequent primary hepatocellular carcinoma

4.56 Causes of unconjugated hyperbilirubinaemia include

　　A cephalhaematoma
　　B hereditary spherocytosis
　　C total parenteral nutrition
　　D meconium plug
　　E breast feeding

4.57 **Lyme disease**

   A is caused by the spirochaete *Borrelia burgdorferi*
   B is carried by an infected tick
   C produces the skin rash erythema chronicum migrans
   D causes lymphadenopathy
   E responds to metronidazole

4.58 **A child with infantile spasms**

   A may have tuberous sclerosis
   B typically presents at the age of 4–8 weeks
   C may respond to steroids
   D may respond to vigabatrin
   E has a 3/sec spike-and-wave pattern on EEG

4.59 **Regarding tests of hearing and language**

   A the Edinburgh articulation test concentrates on the production of consonants
   B the distraction hearing test is routinely performed at 18 months
   C the Reynell developmental language scales do not assess comprehension
   D the Kendall toy test may be useful for assessing a child's hearing and language comprehension at 3 years
   E tympanometry is of most value in assessing inner ear problems

4.60 **Factors associated with an increased risk of Down's syndrome include**

   A raised maternal serum α-fetoprotein
   B low maternal serum unconjugated oestriol
   C high maternal serum human chorionic gonadotrophin
   D multiple pregnancy
   E maternal balanced translocation of chromosome 21 on to chromosome 14

PRACTICE PAPER FIVE

Allow 2 hours for the completion of all 60 questions
Answers are on page 111

5.1 **Acute hemiplegia is a recognized complication of**

    A sickle cell anaemia
    B rubella
    C fracture of the femur
    D mastoiditis
    E systemic lupus erythematosis

5.2 **Organic causes of recurrent abdominal pain include**

    A hydronephrosis
    B lead poisoning
    C school bullying
    D Crohn's disease
    E porphyria

5.3 **In the treatment of childhood asthma**

    A prophylaxis should be considered if β_2-agonists are required more than three times per week
    B inhaler devices are unsuitable for children under the age of 5 years
    C large volume spacer devices enhance deposition of inhaled steroids in the lungs
    D prescription of an inadequate dose is the most common reason for failure of inhaled drugs
    E nebulized β_2-agonists may cause paradoxical bronchoconstriction in children under 18 months of age

5.4 **Burns are**

    A the second commonest cause of accidental death in childhood
    B described as first-degree if the epidermis is destroyed but the dermis is spared
    C painless if the dermis is destroyed
    D classed as major if >10% of the body surface area is affected
    E assessed initially using the rule of fives

5.5 Common causes of pneumonia in an immunocompetent child include

    A *Streptococcus pneumoniae*
    B *Staphylococcus epidermidis*
    C *Haemophilus influenzae*
    D *Mycoplasma pneumoniae*
    E *Pneumocystis carinii*

5.6 The Education Act 1981

    A followed the Calman report
    B states that children should be educated in mainstream schools wherever possible
    C stipulates that a statement of special educational needs can be performed without parental consent
    D gives the parents 60 days to appeal against their child's statement of special educational needs
    E declares that statements should be reviewed on a 3-yearly basis

5.7 The following are features of typical haemolytic uraemic syndrome

    A aplastic anaemia
    B thrombocytopenia
    C hypocalcaemia
    D hypotension
    E prodromal diarrhoeal illness

5.8 Aetiological factors for cerebral palsy include

    A placental abruption
    B hydrocephalus
    C meningitis
    D neonatal hyperbilirubinaemia
    E head injury

5.9 Autism

    A is more common in girls
    B is usually inherited as an autosomal recessive condition
    C may occur in tuberous sclerosis
    D has features which are usually prominent by 9–12 months of life
    E is associated with severe learning difficulties in 95% of children

5.10 Predisposing factors for birth injuries include

   A precipitate delivery
   B cephalic presentation
   C macrosomia
   D twin delivery
   E prematurity

5.11 Clinical features of Patau's syndrome (trisomy 13) include

   A cleft lip and palate
   B rocker bottom feet
   C polydactyly
   D holoprosencephaly
   E Alzheimer's disease

5.12 Talipes

   A is more common in girls
   B is bilateral in 90% of cases
   C has polyhydramnios as a predisposing factor
   D is more commonly equinovarus than calcaneovalgus
   E is usually correctable with gradual manipulation and adhesive strapping

5.13 The following statistics are correct

   A children under 15 years make up two-thirds of the world's population
   B half the world's children live in developed countries
   C the UK currently has a population of approximately 20 million children
   D in the UK there are approximately 500 000 births/year
   E each family doctor has approximately 200 patients under 15 years

5.14 A 4-year-old should be able to

   A ride a tricycle
   B copy a hexagon
   C do up buttons
   D skip
   E go to the toilet alone

5.15 In the management of diabetic ketoacidosis

    A the fluid deficit should be replaced over 4–6 hours
    B insulin reduces the uptake of potassium into cells
    C an insulin infusion should be commenced at 1.0 unit/kg/hour
    D a bicarbonate infusion should be commenced with the insulin infusion
    E shocked patients should be treated with 10–20 ml/kg of colloid

5.16 Enuresis

    A has a prevalence of 20% at 5 years
    B is more common in girls
    C has an underlying organic pathology in 5% of cases
    D is more common in higher socioeconomic groups
    E often has a positive family history

5.17 Causes of failure to thrive include

    A gastro-oesophageal reflux
    B cerebral palsy
    C skeletal dysplasias
    D poor breast-feeding techniques
    E coeliac disease

5.18 In Werdnig–Hoffmann disease

    A inheritance is autosomal dominant
    B death is usually due to renal failure
    C facial muscles are affected
    D there is increased tone at birth
    E death normally occurs within 18 months

5.19 Cerebrospinal fluid (CSF)

    A is produced by the arachnoid villi
    B production is reduced by acetazolamide
    C pressure is elevated in arrested hydrocephalus
    D is absorbed into the cerebral venous sinuses
    E flows from the lateral ventricles through the foramina of Monro

5.20 MMR vaccine is

    A contra-indicated if there is a previous history of mumps
    B a killed vaccine
    C given at 2, 3 and 4 months of age
    D contra-indicated if a child has egg allergy
    E contra-indicated if a child is on immunosuppressive drugs

5.21 Typical presenting features of a metabolic disorder include

    A cataracts
    B developmental delay
    C hyperglycaemia
    D failure to thrive
    E convulsions

5.22 In bacterial meningitis

    A the mortality is 20% in the UK
    B fluids should be restricted to two-thirds of normal requirements
    C steroids should be used routinely in meningococcal meningitis
    D the aetiological agent is usually *Haemophilus influenzae* in the neonatal period
    E ampicillin is the drug of choice in the older age group

5.23 In Duchenne muscular dystrophy

    A genetic mutations can be identified in about 10% of cases
    B the creatinine phosphokinase (CPK) level rises as the disease progresses
    C presentation is usually at 7–10 years
    D inheritance is sex-linked dominant
    E the level of dystrophin correlates with clinical severity

5.24 With regard to the aetiology of osteomyelitis

    A the most common causative organism in the acute case is *Haemophilus influenzae*
    B *Mycobacterium tuberculosis* usually causes chronic osteomyelitis
    C *Salmonella* infection is associated with sickle cell anaemia
    D Group B haemolytic streptococcus is an important cause in neonates
    E *Candida albicans* is implicated in immunosuppressed patients

5.25 In poisoning contra-indications to emesis include

    A consumption of a corrosive substance
    B tinnitus
    C decreased level of consciousness
    D sweating
    E ingestion of a volatile substance

5.26 In pauciarticular juvenile chronic arthritis

    A there is an association with HLA-DRW 5/8
    B chronic iridocyclitis is a major problem
    C systemic symptoms are severe
    D the antinuclear antibody is usually positive
    E the usual age of onset is 5–10 years

5.27 Conditions with autosomal recessive inheritance include

    A oro-facial-digital syndrome
    B cystic fibrosis
    C Becker muscular dystrophy
    D tuberous sclerosis
    E sickle cell disease

5.28 Risk factors for sudden infant death syndrome include

    A supine sleeping position
    B prematurity
    C older maternal age
    D lack of breast feeding
    E maternal smoking

5.29 Upper respiratory tract infections

    A are more common if the parents smoke
    B affect the average child 8–10 times per year
    C are most commonly due to bacterial pathogens
    D may be complicated by feeding disturbance
    E may be of increased severity in overcrowded conditions

5.30 **Squints**

   A are usually incomitant in children
   B affect 10% of children
   C prevent binocular vision
   D if manifest are detected by the cover test
   E if latent may be noticeable when tired

5.31 **In severe combined immunodeficiency**

   A the tonsils are usually hypertrophic
   B mucocutaneous candidiasis is a presenting feature
   C enterovirus infections are frequently fatal
   D bone marrow transplantation offers a long-term cure
   E graft-versus-host disease may be triggered by blood transfusions

5.32 **Regarding herpes simplex virus infection**

   A infection of the neonate affects 2 per 1000 live births in the UK
   B active primary infection at term is an indication for delivery by Caesarean section
   C skin scars on the baby may indicate intra-uterine infection
   D perinatal transmission to the neonate has a high mortality
   E diagnosis can be confirmed by electron microscopy of the vesicle fluid

5.33 **Laboratory features of HIV infection in infants include**

   A hypergammaglobulinaemia
   B thrombocytopenia
   C polycythaemia
   D low CD4 numbers
   E neutropenia

5.34 **Complications of rotavirus gastroenteritis include**

   A acute renal failure
   B cow's milk protein enteropathy
   C sigmoid volvulus
   D hypernatraemia
   E ataxia

5.35 **Breast milk**

   A foremilk has a higher fat content than the hindmilk
   B contains lactoferrin
   C protects the preterm infant against necrotizing enterocolitis
   D contains secretory IgA
   E can be supplemented with human milk fortifiers for preterm infants

5.36 **Recognized features of cyanotic congenital heart disease in childhood include**

   A clubbing
   B thromboembolic events
   C anaemia of chronic disease
   D small stature
   E squatting after exertion

5.37 **Constitutional delay in growth and puberty is associated with**

   A short stature
   B low growth velocity for pubertal stage
   C delayed bone age
   D poor final height prognosis
   E truncal obesity

5.38 **Long-term effects of treatment for childhood leukaemia include**

   A growth impairment
   B precocious puberty
   C delayed puberty
   D cardiotoxicity
   E infertility

5.39 **Ventricular fibrillation is**

   A rare in childhood
   B sometimes seen following near-drowning
   C treated with a first DC shock of 2 J/kg
   D treated with i.v. adrenaline 10 µg/kg prior to any DC shocks
   E sometimes responsive to a precordial thump if the onset is witnessed

5.40 β-thalassaemia major is

   A due to impaired β-globin chain synthesis
   B associated with a low concentration of fetal haemoglobin
   C usually asymptomatic until adolescence
   D more common in children of Afro-Caribbean origin
   E managed with regular blood transfusions

5.41 Slipped femoral epiphysis

   A has a peak age of 5–10 years
   B is due to slippage of the capital epiphysis downwards and backwards
   C is associated with precocious puberty
   D presents with swelling of the hip and thigh
   E is bilateral in 50% of cases

5.42 Hypercalcaemia in childhood

   A is more common than hypocalcaemia
   B is found in association with some renal tumours
   C stimulates parathyroid hormone secretion
   D increases calcitonin secretion
   E may present with failure to thrive

5.43 In idiopathic thrombocytopenic purpura

   A the platelet count returns to normal within 3 months in 75% of cases
   B the risk of intracranial haemorrhage is ~20%
   C bone marrow aspiration should be performed in all cases
   D reduced numbers of megakaryocytes are seen in the bone marrow aspirate
   E systemic lupus erythematosis should be excluded if thrombocytopenia persists for > 6 months

5.44 Wilms' tumour

   A typically presents over the age of 7 years
   B often presents with haematuria
   C has an overall 5-year survival rate of > 70%
   D is associated with heterochromia of the irises
   E is associated with Beckwith–Wiedeman syndrome

5.45 In congenital heart disease

   A   pulmonary stenosis usually presents with an asymptomatic murmur
   B   the murmur associated with an atrial septal defect arises directly from left-to-right flow of blood through the defect
   C   a patent ductus arteriosus is more common in infants who were born prematurely
   D   spontaneous closure of an atrial septal defect is usual
   E   pertussis immunization is contra-indicated

5.46 Clinical features of measles include

   A   conjunctivitis
   B   dry cough
   C   Koplik's spots on the buccal mucosa
   D   incubation period of 14–21 days
   E   maculopapular rash

5.47 Meckel's diverticulum

   A   is a remnant of the embryonic vitello-intestinal duct
   B   may cause profuse rectal bleeding
   C   inflammation may mimic acute appendicitis
   D   is associated with perioral pigmentation
   E   may be the cause of an ileo-ileal intussusception

5.48 Hepatitis A infection

   A   is spread by the faecal-oral route
   B   may be spread antenatally from mother to fetus
   C   leads to a chronic carrier state in 10% of cases
   D   is a cause of aplastic anaemia
   E   may lead to prolonged cholestasis

5.49 Features of biliary atresia include

   A   autosomal dominant inheritance
   B   association with situs inversus
   C   spontaneous haemorrhage
   D   dysmorphic features
   E   white stools

5.50 Complications of Epstein–Barr virus infection are

   A hepatitis
   B acute renal failure
   C splenic rupture
   D thrombocytopenia
   E encephalitis

5.51 Mongolian patches

   A do not occur in Caucasian races
   B persist into adult life
   C are associated with spina bifida occulta
   D may be confused with traumatic bruising
   E are at risk of malignant change

5.52 Chronic ataxia may be caused by

   A aqueduct stenosis
   B metachromatic leucodystrophy
   C hypertension
   D HIV encephalopathy
   E cerebral palsy

5.53 Features of incontinentia pigmenti are

   A autosomal recessive inheritance
   B linear vesicular rash in the neonate
   C the rash fades by adulthood
   D ocular abnormalities
   E polycystic kidneys

5.54 Gastro-intestinal pathogens causing chronic diarrhoea include

   A hookworm
   B *Cryptosporidium parvum*
   C *Giardia lamblia*
   D *Helicobacter pylori*
   E *Yersinia enterocolitica*

5.55 Complications of cystic fibrosis include

    A night blindness
    B portal hypertension
    C arthropathy
    D chronic sinusitis
    E rectal polyps

5.56 Recognized causes of seizures in childhood include

    A breath holding
    B hyponatraemia
    C tuberous sclerosis
    D herpes simplex virus
    E hypocalcaemia

5.57 In the management of constipation

    A lactulose is a stool softener
    B laxatives are rarely needed for more than 3 months
    C senna is a stimulant laxative
    D docusate sodium is a stimulant laxative
    E behaviour problems surrounding toileting are common

5.58 In the assessment of a deaf child

    A microscopic haematuria is associated with Pendred's syndrome
    B heterochromia of the irises is seen in Waardenburg's syndrome
    C a long QT interval on ECG is seen in Lange-Nielsen syndrome
    D rubella specific IgM can be detected until the age of 6 years in congenital rubella
    E a cause can be identified in > 50% of cases

5.59 Developmental warning signs include

    A loss of previously acquired skills
    B inability to walk independently by the age of 12 months
    C hand preference at 5 months
    D Moro reflex persistent at 6 months
    E nystagmus at 3 months

5.60 Causes of hypoglycaemia in childhood include

A alcohol ingestion
B nesidioblastosis
C Rett's syndrome
D septo-optic dysplasia
E Munchausen by proxy

PRACTICE PAPER SIX
Data interpretation and grey case questions

Answers are on page 119

6.1 A 10-day-old baby presents with vomiting and lethargy. His birth weight was 3.6 kg and his weight on admission is 3.1 kg. Initial blood results include: Hb 18.3 g/dl, wbc 10.7×10^9/l, plt 420×10^9/l, Na 123 mmol/l, K 7.6 mmol/l, Bic 20 mmol/l, U 16.4 mmol/l, Cr 63 µmol/l, bilirubin 103 µmol/l, albumin 37 g/l, glu 1.2 mmol/l

A What is the likely diagnosis?
B What investigation would you do to confirm this?
C What is the immediate management?

6.2 A 5-year-old boy presents with bruising. He has been unwell for the preceeding week with coryza and cough. Examination reveals widespread purpura and bruising, a few enlarged cervical lymph nodes but no hepatosplenomegaly. His full blood count is: Hb 10.7 g/dl, wbc 6.3×10^9/l (lymphocytes 5.7, neutrophils 0.6), plt 18×10^9/l

A What is the most likely diagnosis?
B Give three important further investigations?

6.3 A 13-year-old girl is referred to a paediatrician by her school nurse because she is small. Her general health is good. On examination her height is 135 cm (<0.4th centile), weight 29.8 kg (0.4th centile). Her blood pressure is 140/90 on repeated measurements but otherwise general examination is normal. She is pubertal stage 1. Baseline blood tests including full blood count, renal function and liver function tests are normal

A What two further pieces of information should you obtain from her parents or the school nurse?
B Give three important further investigations
C Why might she be hypertensive?

6.4 A 7-year-old boy has been vomiting intermittently for 2 days. Over the last few hours he has become increasingly drowsy. Initial blood tests reveal: Hb 13.6 g/dl, wbc 22.1 × 10⁹/l, plt 371 × 10⁹/l, Na 133 mmol/l, K 4.1 mmol/l, Bic 8 mmol/l, U 17 mmol/l, Cr 77 μmol/l, glu 46 mmol/l

    A What is the diagnosis?
    B Give four important aspects of your initial clinical examination
    C What would be your initial management of this boy?
    D Give two life-threatening complications of the acute management of this condition

6.5 The parents of a nine-month-old boy are at the end of their tether as he has been screaming and irritable for the last 12 hours. He has no past medical history apart from being 'colicky' until he was 6 months old. He has not had his bowels open for 2 days. On examination his fontanelle is mildly sunken and he has dry mucous membranes but he seems settled and happy. During examination of his abdomen he becomes distressed and pale, drawing up his legs in pain. An ill-defined mass is palpable in the right hypochondrium

    A What further clinical information may help you establish the cause of this distress?
    B Give two initial investigations you would perform
    C What is the likely diagnosis?
    D How would you manage this condition?

6.6 A 2½-year-old girl with congenital hypothyroidism, which was picked up on neonatal screening, is currently on thyroxine 75 mcg daily. Her recent thyroid function results are: free thyroxine (FT4) 19.1 pmol/l (normal range 9–23), thyroid stimulating hormone (TSH) 12.4 mU/l (normal range 0.3–5.0).

    A What is the most likely explanation for these results?

6.7 You are asked to see a baby on the postnatal ward at the age of 20 hours who is centrally cyanosed. The oxygen saturation is 37%, the respiratory rate is 40 breaths per minute and the baby is feeding well

A What is the most likely diagnosis?
B What would you expect to hear on auscultation of the praecordium?

On admission to the neonatal unit an ECG is performed which shows left ventricular hypertrophy, right atrial hypertrophy and a QRS axis of +340° (or −20°)

C What is now the likely diagnosis?
D What medical intervention might you consider to improve the baby's oxygen saturation?

6.8 You are called to see a 4-year-old boy who has been an in-patient with offensive diarrhoea for the last 3 days. There has been intermittent blood and mucous in his diarrhoea since admission. The nurses are concerned that he has not passed urine all day. On examination he looks pale but has moist mucous membranes and normal skin turgor. His temperature is 37.6°C, his pulse is 130 bpm, and his blood pressure is 135/90. He has a soft systolic murmur which was not noted on admission and his abdomen is generally tender

A What is the likely diagnosis?
B How would you confirm the diagnosis?
C Why might he have developed a murmur?

6.9 The parents of a 7-year-old girl have noticed the growth of pubic hair over the last 3 months. On examination her height is 122 cm (91st centile), weight 23 kg (75th centile), she has no breast development (Tanner stage 1), and sparse pigmented pubic hairs chiefly along the labia (Tanner stage 2)

A Give three other aspects of her clinical examination which are important in identifying the likely cause
B Give four investigations which might be indicated

6.10 A 5-year-old girl has developed marked generalized oedema over the last 3 days. She is now complaining of abdominal pain and is refusing to eat or drink. Dipstick urinalysis reveals proteinuria 4+ and haematuria 3+. Her blood pressure is 130/75 and initial investigations reveal: Hb 15.1g/dl, wbc 7.3 × 10^9/l, plt 476 × 10^9/l, Na 135 mmol/l, K 4.9 mmol/l, U 8.7 mmol/l, Cr 106 µmol/l, albumin 9 g/l, urinary Na undetectable, urinary protein excretion 10.7 g/24h

   A What is the diagnosis?
   B Give two possible causes for her abdominal pain
   C What information does the undetectable urinary sodium give you?

6.11 A 2-year-old boy has had an intermittent fever for the last 6 days. On examination his temperature is 38.9°C, he is miserable and lethargic. He has bilateral conjunctivitis and a few enlarged cervical lymph nodes. His lips are dry and cracked and he has a widespread faint macular rash. His blood pressure is 100/60 and his chest is clear. He has no hepatosplenomegaly. His parents feel that his hands and feet are a little swollen

   A What is the likely diagnosis?
   B How would you confirm the diagnosis?
   C What treatment should he receive?
   D What is the prognosis?

6.12 A 4-week-old baby is referred with prolonged jaundice. He was born at full term, birth weight 3.1 kg and he has been breast feeding well. On examination his liver is palpable 2 cm below the costal margin, but the rest of the examination is unremarkable. The mother's blood group is A positive and the baby's blood group is O positive. His urine is rather dark and tests positive for bilirubin.

   A What is the most important initial investigation?
   B Give two immediate complications of which the baby is at risk
   C Give two important differential diagnoses

6.13 A 2-year-old caucasian boy is referred with short stature. His length followed the 9th centile from birth to approximately 1 year of age. It has now fallen to below the 0.4th centile. Developmentally he has progressed normally and he started walking independently at the age of 14 months. His mother is 4'6" and his father is 5'10". On examination his weight is 10.8 kg (9th centile) and his sitting height is on the 25th centile. He walks with a waddling gait and he has marked bowing of his legs. Investigation results include: total serum calcium 2.24 mmol/l (normal range 2.2–2.75), serum phosphate 0.56 mmol/l (normal range 1.16–1.91), serum alkaline phosphatase 1020 U/l (normal range 100–850), plasma parathyroid hormone level normal

    A What is the most likely diagnosis?
    B This boy has a younger sister aged 4 months, is she likely to suffer with the same condition?

6.14 A baby was delivered by emergency caesarian section for foetal bradycardia. She cried on delivery and looked pink but was transferred to the neonatal unit as she remained bradycardic with a heart rate of 42 bpm. Investigations revealed: Chest X-ray normal, ECG narrow QRS complex, atrial rate 135/min, ventricular rate 42/min

    A What is the diagnosis?
    B What investigation would you perform on her mother?

6.15 A distressed 15-year-old girl arrives in casualty by ambulance complaining of difficulty breathing. Arterial blood gases breathing 28% oxygen are: pH 7.66, pCO_2 2.2 kPa, pO_2 22.0 kPa, Bic 20 mmol/l

    A What does the blood gas show?
    B What is the most likely cause?

6.16 A child can (1) say 20 clear words; (2) do a circular scribble in imitation; (3) creep on her hands and knees

    A Comment on this child's development

6.17 An 18-month-old boy is referred to the paediatric department as his GP is worried about the number of bruises he has on his limbs. His health visitor is concerned about non-accidental injury. Investigations reveal:
Hb 12.2 g/dl, wbc 5.1 × 10⁹/l, plt 256 × 10⁹/l, prothrombin time 12 sec (control 12 sec), partial thromboplastin time 130 sec (control 45 sec), thrombin time 17 sec (control 18 sec)

A What is the differential diagnosis?
B What further investigations should be performed?

6.18 The following is the pedigree of a family with an inherited condition in which the affected individuals have learning difficulties and distinctive craniofacial features.

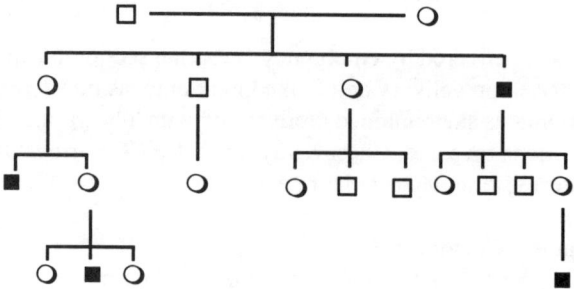

☐ unaffected male
○ unaffected female
■ affected male
● affected female

A What is the inheritance pattern?
B What is the condition most likely to be?

6.19 A baby with a cleft lip and palate is reviewed at the age of 6 weeks. She is noted to be pale and generally listless. Her mother says that she is not interested in feeding. Investigations show: Hb 4.2 g/dl, wbc 12.1 × 10⁹/l, plt 237 × 10⁹/l, MCV 97, reticulocytes <0.5%, film – normochromic with mild macrocytosis. On the basis of these results bone marrow aspiration is performed and this shows virtual absence of nucleated red cell precursors.

A What is the diagnosis?

6.20 A 6-week-old baby presents with vomiting and poor feeding. His weight was on the 50th centile at birth but is now on the 3rd centile. On examination he is noted to have hepatosplenomegaly and bilateral cataracts. Urine testing shows a positive reaction with Clinitest® (Bayer Diagnostics) and a negative reaction with Clinistix® (Bayer Diagnostics)

    A What do the two tests indicate?
    B What is the likely diagnosis?
    C What treatment is required?

6.21 An 8-year-old boy with a heart murmur is under regular review in the cardiology clinic. In the past he was investigated for failure to thrive and severe constipation at the age of 8 weeks and was found to be hypercalcaemic. This resolved and since then his general health has been good. He has moderate learning difficulties, prominent lips, an upturned nose, and low set ears

    A What is the most likely diagnosis?
    B What is the cardiac defect likely to be?

6.22 The following results are obtained on cardiac catheterization:

Site	O2 saturation (%)	Pressure (mmHg)
SVC	62	
RA	63	5
RV	65	92
IVC	65	
PA	65	19/8
LA	98	7
LV	90	90
Aorta	85	90/58

    A What is the likely diagnosis?

6.23 A 22-year-old women, who is fit and healthy, gives birth to a baby with Down's syndrome. The mother's karyotype is checked and the result is reported as 45 XX, t (14,21)

    A How would you interpret this result?
    B What advice would you give her with regard to the risk of Down's syndrome affecting future pregnancies?

6.24 An infant born at 27 week's gestation weighing 730 g is ventilated from birth for respiratory distress syndrome. The ventilator settings are as follows: peak inspiratory pressure 22 mmHg, positive end expiratory pressure 4 mmHg, inspiratory time 0.45 sec, rate 60 breaths per minute, inspired oxygen concentration 63%.

At the age of 4 hours arterial blood gas analysis shows pH 7.34, pO_2 8.9 kPa, pCO_2 5.6 kPa, base excess –3.4

The baby subsequently receives a dose of artificial surfactant via the endotracheal tube and the oxygen requirements fall to 45% over the next 2 hours.

At the age of 9 hours the baby is noted to be a poor colour and the oxygen requirements have risen to 75% over the last 30 minutes. Arterial blood gas analysis reveals: pH 7.19, pO_2 5.3 kPa, pCO_2 8.6 kPa, base excess –9.3

A What does the second blood gas show?
B Give two possible explanations for the deterioration and explain how you would manage them

6.25 A 3-year-old girl is referred to outpatients with poor weight gain. Her birth weight was 3.47 kg (50th centile) and subsequent weights followed the 25th centile until the age of 6 months. Since then she has gradually fallen to below the 0.4th centile. She is described as a picky eater, her stools are intermittently loose, and she has become increasingly lethargic over the last 9 months. On examination her height is 87 cm (2nd centile), weight 9.87 kg (<0.4th centile), she looks thin, pale and miserable. Her abdomen is a little distended but there is no organomegaly. Investigations reveal: Hb 7.9 g/dl, MCV 67, wbc 7 × 10⁹/l, plt 376 × 10⁹/l, ferritin 6 ng/ml (normal range 15–100), Na 142 mmol/l, K 3.9 mmol/l, U 5.3 mmol/l, albumin 29 g/l. Stool for ova, cysts, parasites and culture negative.

A What is the likely diagnosis?
B How would you confirm the diagnosis?
C What treatment is required?

ANSWERS TO PAPER ONE

The correct answers appear in bold
The topic names given in brackets refer to the topics in *Key Topic in Paediatrics*

1.1 **B C E** (Acute renal failure)
    A diuretics will worsen hypovolaemia
    D may result in obstructive uropathy due to uric acid crystals

1.2 **C D E** (Adrenal disorders)
    A autosomal recessive
    B 21-hydroxylase deficiency resulting in accumulation of 17-hydroxyprogesterone

1.3 **A E** (Anaemia)
    B this is the normal time to introduce solids – iron deficiency anaemia is associated with late weaning especially if purely breast fed
    C early introduction of doorstep cow's milk may cause microscopic gastrointestinal bleeding. Formula milk is recommended until 12 months
    D does cause a marked microcytic hypochromic anaemia but should not be confused with iron deficiency

1.4 **B** (Arrhythmias)
    A uncommon
    C usually 220–300 bpm
    D vagal manoeuvres and drugs (e.g. adenosine) should be tried first if stable
    E slows conduction through the atrioventricular node

1.5 **A C E** (Calcium metabolism)
    B is suppressed by hypercalcaemia
    D increases phosphate excretion

1.6 **D E** (Cardiopulmonary resuscitation)
    A chin lift with the head in the neutral position
    B one finger breadth below the nipple line
    C brachial or femoral artery – the relatively short fat neck of an infant makes the carotids difficult to feel

1.7 **B D E** (Chronic renal failure)
    A microcytic anaemia
    C type IV hyperlipidaemia

1.8 **A B C** (Coma)
  D may lead to an arrhythmia but does not directly cause acute encephalopathy
  E causes nausea, vomiting and irritability but not an acute encephalopathy

1.9 **B E** (Congenital heart disease – acyanotic)
  A acyanotic in 70% of cases
  C approximately 50% of children with Down's syndrome have congenital heart disease
  D no association

1.10 **A B C E** (Chromosomal abnormalities)
  D increased risk of glue ear with a high incidence of conductive deafness

1.11 **C D** (Diabetes mellitus)
  A a random glucose of > 11mmol/l confirms the diagnosis. A glucose tolerance test is rarely indicated
  B more common with increasing distance from the equator
  E rare at presentation

1.12 **B D** (Enuresis)
  A only 1–2%
  C drug therapy is inappropriate before ~7 years at the earliest, and only if other management strategies (e.g. reward systems) have failed
  E 1% still wet at 15 years and a small number still wet as adults

1.13 **B** (Glomerulonephritis)
  Glomerulonephritis is associated with sensorineural deafness in Alport's syndrome
  A sometimes described as 'smokey' – frothy urine associated with heavy proteinuria
  C C3 and C4 levels fall in post-streptococcal glomerulonephritis and lupus nephritis
  D only if the renal function is rapidly deteriorating or renal impairment persists for several weeks
  E uncommon

1.14 **B** (Growth – short and tall stature)
   A not reliably – the use and interpretation of stimulation tests is controversial
   C GH insufficiency is rare. Consider other more common causes of growth failure first (i.e. inadequate nutrition, chronic illness, Turner's syndrome)
   D daily subcutaneous injections
   E low IGF-1 levels

1.15 **A D** (Haematuria)
   B cystinuria
   C associated with nephrocalcinosis (deposition of calcium in the renal parenchyma)
   E no increased risk

1.16 **C D** (Children and the law)
   A lasts for up to 8 days but may be challenged after 72 hours
   B emergency protection order used in these cases
   E decides what contact the child may have with other people

1.17 **C D** (Haemophilia and Christmas disease)
   A less severe
   B factor IX precipitates are given for acute bleeds, but no regular treatment is given
   E sex-linked recessive

1.18 **A D E** (Heart failure)
   B tachycardia
   C symptoms tend to worsen as pulmonary vascular resistance falls over the first 6 weeks of life

1.19 **B D E** (Cleft lip and palate)
   A more common in boys (3M:2F)
   C more common on the left

1.20 **C D E** (Leukaemia and lymphoma)
   A <5% at diagnosis
   B best diagnosed by examination of CSF for leukaemic blasts. A CT scan may be required prior to LP if there are concerns about raised intracranial pressure

1.21 **B C E** (Developmental assessment)
   A, D these would be expected at 18 months

1.22 **B D E** (Neonatal respiratory distress)
A ~20% of babies <2.5 kg develop RDS
C prolonged rupture of the membranes tends to advance fetal maturation and decrease the severity of RDS

1.23 **B C D E** (Neonatal surgery)
A seems to have a protective effect

1.24 **A B** (Nephrotic syndrome)
C rarely indicated
D increased clotting tendency
E >75% will have at least one relapse and these are usually steroid responsive. Cyclophosphamide is considered if frequently relapsing or the side effects of steroids become unacceptable (e.g. growth suppression)

1.25 **C D** (Polyuria and renal tubular disorders)
A rises to >750 mosmol/l in normal subjects
B unresponsive to DDAVP, cf. central diabetes insipidus
E usually high

1.26 **A C E** (Prematurity)
B no racial differences
D poor socioeconomic background

1.27 **A C D E** (Puberty – precocious and delayed)
B LH stimulates release of testosterone, FSH stimulates spermatogenesis

1.28 **D E** (Purpura and bruising)
A rash is the first symptom in >50%
B microscopic haematuria occurs in >70%
C clotting studies are normal

1.29 **A C D** (Peripheral neuropathy)
B microcytic anaemia
E raised

1.30 **A B C D E** (Small for gestational age, large for gestational age)

1.31 **A B D** (Acute hemiplegia)
C progressive arterial occlusion
E small artery occlusion

1.32 **B D** (Lower respiratory tract infection)
- A 3–4 yearly intervals
- C absolute lymphocytosis
- E given as part of the triple vaccine at 2, 3, and 4 months

1.33 **B E** (Allergy)
- A type 1 is immediate hypersensitivity (anaphylactic) reaction
- C type 4 is delayed or cell-mediated hypersensitivity
- D type 2 is cytotoxic reaction

1.34 **A B D E** (Behaviour)
- C there is poor attachment to parents

1.35 **B D** (Congenital heart disease – cyanotic)
- A excludes a major right-to-left shunt (some cardiologists say > 20 kPa)
- C suggestive of tricuspid atresia
- E prostaglandin E2 is used to maintain duct patency – indomethacin is used to close the duct

1.36 **B D E** (Drowning and near-drowning)
- A raised ICP may develop
- C hypothermia is usual

1.37 **A B D E** (Dysmorphology and teratogenesis)
- C recommended during pregnancy to reduce the risk of neural tube defects

1.38 **A D** (Inborn errors of metabolism)
- B organic acid disorder
- C urea cycle defect
- E disorder of carbohydrate metabolism

1.39 **A B D** (Polyarthritis)
- C, E these are minor features

1.40 **A C E** (Upper respiratory tract infection)
- B may be a factor in chronic sinusitis but is not in itself an indication for adenotonsillectomy
- D recurrent tonsillitis may be

1.41 **A C** (Coeliac disease)
- B the presence of circulating antibodies is an adjunct to assessment but is not diagnostic
- D barium follow-through is often non-specifically abnormal, but not routinely performed
- E ESPGAN 1989 criteria for diagnosis

1.42 **A D** (Abdominal pain – acute)
- B Crohn's disease usually causes recurrent abdominal pain
- C leucocytes in the urine occur in appendicitis, UTI, and many other systemic infections
- E mesenteric adenitis is usually viral in origin

1.43 **A B C E** (Neurocutaneous syndromes)
- D calcification is typically found after the first year of life

1.44 **A B D E** (Eczema)
- C the groin area is more usually affected in infantile seborrhoeic dermatitis

1.45 **B C E** (Kawasaki disease)
- A no definite pathogen or vector yet implicated
- D prevalence in the UK is 3 per 100 000

1.46 **A B E** (Stridor)
- C usually pre-school children, typically during the second year of life
- D restlessness indicates hypoxia with severe upper airways obstruction

1.47 **A B D E** (Immunodeficiency)
- C this is typical of IgG-2 subclass deficiency

1.48 **A B C E** (Lymphadenopathy)
- D the lymph nodes are not usually enlarged

1.49 **A C D E** (Liver disease)
- B a papular dermatitis may occur in acute hepatitis B infection but is not a specific feature of fulminant hepatic failure

1.50 **B D E** (Congenital infection)
- A the organism is a Gram-positive rod
- C intra-uterine growth retardation is not a feature

1.51 **A B D E** (Vomiting)
- C barium studies are of use to detect anatomical lesions, but 24 hour oesophageal pH monitoring is currently the method of choice for the diagnosis of reflux

1.52 **A B C E** (HIV infection)
- D there is no definite evidence that delivery by Caesarean section reduces transmission rates

1.53 **B C** (Gastroenteritis)
- A breast feeding should continue throughout the illness
- D antidiarrhoeal agents do not reduce fluid losses and have serious side-effects
- E acidosis normally self-corrects with improved tissue perfusion after rehydration

1.54 **B C E** (Nutrition)
- A with complete rest small bowel and pancreatic atrophy may occur
- D a fall in platelet count may indicate catheter sepsis but is not a contraindication to TPN

1.55 **A B C E** (Single gene defects)
- D X-linked dominant

1.56 **B E** (Cerebral palsy)
- A cerebral palsy is non-progressive. The disability may become more obvious with age as more milestones are not achieved and the predominant disorder of movement may change (e.g. neonatal hypotonia and then increasing spasticity with age) but the underlying brain damage does not progress
- C ~2 per 1000
- D has a clear aetiological factor in less than one-third of cases

1.57 **A C D E** (Blistering conditions)
- B palatal petechiae and a macular rash may occur, not blistering

1.58 **B C D** (Chronic diarrhoea)
- A nocturnal diarrhoea indicates significant pathology, and is not a feature of toddler diarrhoea in which the first stool of the day is often formed
- E constipation predisposes children to urinary tract infections

1.59 **C D E** (Seizures)
- A 3–5%
- B this is a complex febrile convulsion

1.60 **A B C D** (Rashes and naevi)
- E nail changes sometimes associated with chronic psoriasis but not guttate psoriasis

ANSWERS TO PAPER TWO

The correct answers appear in bold
The topic names in brackets refer to the topics in *Key Topics in Paediatrics*

2.1 **A C** (Acute renal failure)
   B suggests a pre-renal cause (e.g. hypovolaemia)
   D given orally or rectally to increase elimination of potassium from the body
   E dilutional hyponatraemia may occur

2.2 **C D E** (Adrenal disorders)
   A the most common cause is corticosteroid treatment (i.e. exogenous glucocorticoid)
   B Cushing's *disease*

2.3 **None true** (Anaemia)
   A autosomal dominant
   B negative
   C anaemia is variable and transfusions are needed infrequently
   D fava beans precipitate haemolysis in G6PD deficiency
   E delay as long as possible due to risk of infections (e.g. pneumococcal)

2.4 **A C D E** (Arrhythmias)
   B the Wenckebach phenomenon is a type of second-degree heart block, complete AV dissociation is described as third-degree heart block

2.5 **A D** (Calcium metabolism)
   B secondary hyperparathyroidism, acidosis, relative vitamin D resistance (*see* Chronic renal failure)
   C inadequate phosphate intake
   E increased renal phosphate loss

2.6 **A E** (Cardiopulmonary resuscitation)
   B poor prognosis due to generalized tissue hypoxia prior to the cardiac arrest
   C secure the airway and adequately ventilate before giving any drugs
   D DC shock is used in ventricular fibrillation

2.7 **A B D** (Chronic renal failure)
   C symptomatic uraemia despite conservative treatment is an indication
   E indicates significant renal impairment but is not in itself an indication for dialysis

2.8   **B C** (Coma)
       A   decorticate posture
       D   <u>A</u>irway <u>B</u>reathing <u>C</u>irculation first
       E   may be absent if the intracranial pressure rises rapidly

2.9   **B E** (Congenital heart disease – acyanotic)
       A   these are features of an innocent murmur
       C   left to right
       D   >50% close spontaneously

2.10   **A C D** (Developmental assessment)
       B, E   these are milestones at 3 months

2.11   **C E** (Diabetes mellitus)
       A   there is often an increased insulin requirement during an intercurrent illness despite a decreased food intake
       B   finger prick blood sugars
       D   there is relative insulin resistance due to increased GH secretion during puberty

2.12   **B D** (Enuresis)
       A   there is usually a history of constant dribbling and primary enuresis
       C   rarely indicated
       E   may be due to a psychosocial upset (e.g. change of school) and in these situations reward systems are often helpful

2.13   **A B E** (Glomerulonephritis)
       C   microscopic haematuria commonly persists for 1–2 years with no prognostic significance. If it persists for longer than this, other conditions such as lupus nephritis should be excluded
       D   dialysis is rarely needed

2.14   **B C D** (Growth – short and tall stature)
       A   considerable variability throughout the year
       E   velocity is normal for pubertal stage. There is a steady deceleration in growth rate during childhood which continues until the pubertal growth spurt occurs

2.15   **C E** (Haematuria)
       A   persistent microscopic haematuria with intermittent macroscopic haematuria
       B   rarely the presenting feature. Usually presents as an asymptomatic abdominal mass
       D   >70% of children with HSP have microscopic haematuria

2.16   B D E (Poisoning)
       A   hyperventilation and deep sighing respirations due to a metabolic acidosis
       C   hyperpyrexia, vasodilatation and sweating

2.17   A C (Haemophilia and Christmas disease)
       B   usually mild bleeding problems unless <5% of the normal level
       D   physiotherapy is a vital part of the recovery process to prevent ankylosis
       E   normal

2.18   A B C E (Neonatal convulsions)
       D   the potassium may rise if there is renal impairment

2.19   A C D E (Hypertension)
       B   a child with hypertension may present with headaches, vomiting and visual disturbance so hypertension should be excluded before a diagnosis of migraine is made

2.20   A B C D E (Leukaemia and lymphoma)

2.21   B C D (Inborn errors of metabolism)
       A, E   do not cause hyperammonaemia

2.22   A B C D E (Neonatal respiratory distress)

2.23   A D (Neonatal surgery)
       B   polyhydramnios
       C   >85% but not all
       E   this would suggest the presence of a diaphragmatic hernia

2.24   B E (Nephrotic syndrome)
       A   uncommon, prevalence 6 per 100 000
       C   >90% are steroid responsive
       D   typical of acute nephritic syndrome

2.25   A B E (Polyuria and renal tubular disorders)
       Muscle weakness is due to the hypokalaemia which occurs in distal RTA
       C   failure of the distal tubules to excrete hydrogen ions. Increased bicarbonate loss occurs in proximal RTA
       D   hyperchloraemic, hypokalaemic acidosis

2.26   B C D E (Prematurity)
       A   >70% in most units

2.27 **A D E** (Puberty – precocious and delayed)
B the majority of boys have a pathological cause so they need thorough investigation, cf. girls who usually have idiopathic precocious puberty
C an advanced bone age is usual

2.28 **B C** (Solid tumours)
A > 50% 5-year survival
D most have metastases at presentation
E not currently in the UK, but has been part of a screening programme in Japan

2.29 **A B C E** (Thyroid disorders)
D delayed skeletal maturation is usual

2.30 **A B E** (Urinary tract infection)
C DMSA scans detect renal scarring. The presence of scars may be predictive of the presence of reflux but does not reliably diagnose it
D surgery is required in only a very small proportion of children with reflux

2.31 **C D E** (Acute hemiplegia)
Mycotic aneurysms can develop as a result of subacute bacterial endocarditis leading to a risk of intracranial haemorrhage. Polycystic kidney disease is associated with an increased risk of cerebral aneurysms.
A antithrombin III is the main physiological inhibitor of coagulation. Deficiencey leads to an increased tendency to thrombosis rather than haemorrhage
B there is no increased risk as the platelet count and clotting studies are normal

2.32 **A B D E** (Asthma)
Tachypnoea is usual during an asthma attack and this hyperventilation leads to a low pCO_2. A normal respiratory rate and a normal or raised pCO_2 suggest that the child is becoming exhausted.
C bilateral wheeze is often heard in mild and moderate attacks, a silent chest is more worrying as it suggests very poor air entry

2.33 **A B C D E** (Lower respiratory tract infection)

2.34 **A B D E** (Allergy)
C hypotension occurs

2.35 **A B C D E** (Child abuse)

2.36 **A B E** (Chromosomal abnormalities)
   C these are a feature of Down's syndrome
   D there is an increased risk of leukaemia in Down's syndrome

2.37 **B E** (Congenital dislocation of the hip and talipes)
   A it is treated with an abduction splint
   C the acetabulum is shallow
   D interpretation of radiographs of the unossified hip is difficult

2.38 **A D E** (Ataxia)
   B Tendon reflexes are absent or reduced
   C Friedrich's ataxia is associated with optic atrophy

2.39 **A D** (Meningitis and encephalitis)
   B only close contacts under 5 years who have not been immunized
   C prophylaxis for contacts is not indicated in these cases
   E orange–red discolouration

2.40 **A D E** (Polyarthritis)
   B equally common in boys and girls
   C rheumatoid factor negative

2.41 **B C D** (Vision)
   A only from age 4–5 years
   E test of colour vision

2.42 **D** (Purpura and bruising *and* Gastrointestinal haemorrhage)
   A small haemorrhages into the gut wall are usually responsible for positive faecal occult blood tests
   B lesions are found on extensor surfaces of limbs and buttocks. Lip telangiectasia are found in hereditary haemorrhagic telangiectasia, and perioral pigmentation in Peutz–Jeger syndrome
   C the platelet count and coagulation screen are normal
   E bone marrow examination is not indicated in Henoch–Schönlein purpura. Megakaryocytes are found in the bone marrow of patients with idiopathic thrombocytopaenic purpura (ITP)

2.43 **C E** (Coeliac disease)
   A symptoms occur after a variable period up to 7 years
   B the proximal small bowel is predominantly affected
   D the risk to first degree relatives is 10%

2.44 **B C** (Abdominal pain – acute)
   A typically presents between 6–12 months of age
   D plain abdominal X-ray shows signs of small bowel obstruction, also the soft-tissue shadow of the intussusception
   E barium enema is diagnostic, and hydrostatic reduction by the column of barium may be curative, but barium meal is rarely indicated

2.45 **B C D E** (Constipation)
   A there is incomplete development of ganglion cells in the plexuses of Meissner and Auerbach

2.46 **A B C D** (Neurocutaneous syndromes)
   E Acoustic neuroma is a feature of type 2 neurofibromatosis (NF2)

2.47 **A C** (Eczema)
   B sedatives used for short periods may help break the itch–scratch cycle
   D systemic antibiotics are generally preferable
   E dietary manipulation may be helpful for a minority of patients

2.48 **A B E** (Kawasaki disease)
   C diagnosis requires the exclusion of staphylococcal and streptococcal infection
   D Erythema marginatum is a transient pink rash with raised edges which occurs in rheumatic fever. The rash of Kawasaki disease is polymorphous

2.49 **A D** (Stridor)
   B cough is not prominent
   C typically the child sits forward to relieve the obstruction
   E stridor is usually soft

2.50 **B E** (Immunodeficiency)
   A Hypocalcaemia (hypoparathyroidism) is found
   C Eczema is associated with Wiskott–Aldrich syndrome
   D there are defects of T-cell function

2.51 **A B D** (Lymphadenopathy)
   C generalized lymphadenopathy is caused by phenytoin and carbamazepine
   E lymphadenopathy is not a clinical feature

Lloyd JK. Hyperlipidaemia. *Current Paediatrics*, 1992; **2**: 111–13

2.52 **A B C E** (Liver disease)
  D vitamin D deficiency may arise in chronic liver disease but vitamin D poisoning is not a cause of FHF

Choonara I. Drugs causing liver damage. *Current Paediatrics*, 1995; **5**: 21–3

2.53 **A B E** (Congenital infection)
  C there is greatest risk of fetal damage during the first trimester – up to 90% of pregnancies infected during the first 8–10 weeks are affected
  D there is no specific treatment

2.54 **A C D** (Vomiting)
  B presentation between the 3rd to 8th week of life is typical
  E the thickened pylorus is felt in the right hypochondrium

2.55 **B C** (HIV infection)
  A bilateral reticulonodular infiltrates occur early in the disease, often in the absence of symptoms
  D nebulized pentamidine is used as prophylaxis against *Pneumocystis carinii* pneumonia. It is not used to treat LIP
  E haemoptysis is not a feature of LIP - cough, dyspnoea and hypoxaemia are typical

2.56 **B D E** (Seizures)
  A hyperventilation
  C 3/sec spike-and-wave. Hypsarrhythmia is typical of infantile spasms

2.57 **B C D** (Rashes and naevi *and* Childhood exanthemata)
  A rubella causes a transient pink macular rash
  E there is an erythematous rash, with mucous membrane ulceration

2.58 **A B C D E** (Hearing and speech)

2.59 **A** (Childhood exanthemata)
  B the rash is pink, macular, but transient
  C mucous membrane involvement is not a feature
  D orchitis is a feature of mumps infection
  E jaundice occurs in congenital rubella syndrome

2.60 **A D E** (Cystic fibrosis)
  B levels of immunoreactive trypsin are raised, due to pancreatic damage *in utero*
  C the delta F508 mutation accounts for 70% of CF mutations in northern Europe and North America

ANSWERS TO PAPER THREE

The correct answers appear in bold
The topic names in brackets refer to the topics in *Key Topics in Paediatrics*

3.1 **B C D E** (Acute renal failure)
    A peaked T waves, depressed R waves, prolonged QRS and PR intervals

3.2 **B C** (Adrenal disorders)
    30% of cases of adrenal insufficiency are now thought to be due to adrenoleucodystrophy which can be diagnosed on VLCFAs
    A BP is normal, cf. Conn's syndrome
    D typical of Addison's disease
    E rising potassium

3.3 **A B C** (Growth – short and tall stature)
    D parental heights are corrected for the sex of the child by adding 12.6 cm to the mother's height for a boy or subtracting 12.6 cm from the father's height for a girl (with the new nine centile growth charts a correction factor of 14 cm may be more appropriate)
    E height velocity calculation requires two height measurements separated by as long a period as possible (preferably 1 year)

Freeman JV. *Archives of Disease in Childhood*, 1995; **73**: 17–24

3.4 **C E** (Arrhythmias)
    A transient falls in heart rate are not uncommon especially during sleep
    B uncommon in infancy
    D vagal stimulation (diving reflex)

3.5 **B C** (Calcium metabolism)
    A <1%
    D low
    E low due to hypoalbuminaemia

3.6 **D E** (Poisoning)
    A maximal at 3–4 days post ingestion
    B needs to be given within 12 hours of ingestion
    C can only be given intravenously

3.7 **B C E** (Chronic renal failure)
    Chronic renal failure is associated with sensorineural deafness in Alport's syndrome
    A <5% = end-stage renal failure, chronic renal failure = 5–25%
    D 30–35% secondary to glomerulonephritis

3.8   **A B C D E** (Coma)
Reye's syndrome is an acute encephalopathy associated with fatty degeneration of the liver. The aetiology is obscure but there is a possible association with aspirin ingestion, varicella and influenzae B infections.

3.9   **A B E** (Congenital heart disease – acyanotic)
   C   femoral pulses may be palpable particularly before the ductus arteriosus closes
   D   left ventricular hypertrophy

3.10 **A C E** (Immunization)
   B   a minor infection without pyrexia at the time of vaccination is not a contra-indication
   D   a fever of >39.5°C within 48 hours of a previous immunization is a contra-indication

3.11 **A D** (Ataxia)
   B, C, E   piperazine, phenytoin, thallium, alcohol and solvent abuse are all known to cause ataxia but digoxin, acyclovir and ciprofloxacin do not

3.12 **A C** (Sickle cell anaemia and thalassaemia syndromes)
   B   usually asymptomatic until levels of HbF fall (i.e. about 6 months)
   D   HbSS tends to be more severe
   E   HbF 5–10% in an adult with sickle cell anaemia, whereas it normally represents <5% of the total by 6 months of age

3.13 **B D E** (Glomerulonephritis)
   A   typically affects school-age children
   C   this is a feature of nephrotic syndrome

3.14 **A B C D** (Haemolytic uraemic syndrome)
   E   may cause haemolysis

3.15 **B C** (Blistering conditions)
   A   children under the age of 6 years usually affected
   D   dermatitis herpetiformis is associated with a gluten-sensitive enteropathy
   E   dystrophic epidermolysis bullosa heals with scarring

3.16 **C D E** (Thyroid disorders)
   A   1 in 3000–4000
   B   does not exclude secondary or tertiary hypothyroidism in which TSH is normal or low

Grant DB. *Archives of Disease in Childhood*, 1995; **72**: 85–9

3.17   A C D (Urinary tract infection)
       B twice as common in boys in the neonatal period
       E micturating cystography should be delayed until the urine is clear of infection. Most paediatricians would arrange a cystogram for infants under 1 year of age but there is debate as to whether it is necessary in older children who have normal US and DMSA scans

3.18   A C D E (Childhood exanthemata *and* Congenital infection)
       B other infections are generally responsible for acute post-infectious glomerulonephritis (e.g. Group A beta-haemolytic streptococcus)

3.19   A B E (Shock)
       C originally associated with tampon use but now known also to occur in children with focal staphylococcal infections
       D typically staphylococcal infections – a toxic shock-like syndrome can also be caused by group A haemolytic streptococcus

3.20   B C (Leukaemia and lymphoma)
       A 3 times more common in boys
       D peak incidence 7–10 years
       E 85–90% 5-year survival if localized, but only 30–40% in advanced disease

3.21   A D E (Purpura and bruising)
       B normal platelet count
       C platelet dysfunction, platelet count normal

3.22   A C D (Peripheral neuropathy)
       B no association
       E no association

3.23   None true (Neonatal surgery)
       A rarely, cf. exomphalos major
       B outcome is improved if the baby can be stabilized for at least 12 hours prior to surgery
       C most are managed medically
       D exomphalos 1 in 10 000 – gastroschisis 1 in 6000
       E elective Caesarian section does not improve outcome

3.24   A B D E (Small for gestational age, large for gestational age)
       C usually have less severe RDS

3.25 **C D E** (Polyuria and renal tubular disorders)
   A it is an autosomal recessive condition so there is a 1 in 4 risk of female siblings being affected
   B seen in cystinuria

3.26 **B D** (Prematurity)
   A haemorrhage occurs from the capillaries of the germinal layer
   C 90% occur by day 3
   E limited to germinal layer = grade I IVH, sequelae very uncommon

3.27 **A B** (Puberty – precocious and delayed)
   C associated with precocious puberty
   D used to treat precocious puberty
   E usually constitutional so imaging is indicated only if there are neurological signs or symptoms, cf. precocious puberty in boys

3.28 **A B D E** (Rashes and naevi)
   C itching is not a prominent symptom

3.29 **A B D E** (Limping and joint disorders)
   C typically causes a limp without swelling or pain

3.30 **A B** (Solid tumours)
   C distant metastases are rare
   D 50% arise in the posterior fossa
   E overall only 50% 5-year survival with surgery and radiotherapy even if completely resected – there is a high potential for local recurrence particularly if the histology is high grade

3.31 **A B C D E** (Asthma)

3.32 **A D** (Lower respiratory tract infection)
   B approximately one-third are non-respiratory (e.g. cervical lymphadenitis, TB meningitis)
   C sputum collection is often difficult in children as they tend to swallow it. Other possible ways to make the diagnosis include gastric washings, Mantoux test, bone marrow aspirate, lymph node biopsy
   E is notifiable

3.33 **A B D E** (Demography and definitions)
   C not notifiable but cases have been monitored by the British Paediatric Association surveillance unit

3.34 **A C E** (Child abuse)
   B young mothers
   D first born most at risk

3.35   **E** (Chromosomal abnormalities)
       A the Xq27 folate sensitive fragile site is on the long arm of the X chromosome
       B testes are large particularly after puberty
       C large head often >97th centile
       D usually moderate to severe learning difficulties

3.36   **A C D** (Developmental delay and regression)
       B agenesis of the corpus callosum may be found in a child with global developmental delay but it can be an incidental finding in normal individuals and is not a cause in itself
       E not a cause of developmental delay

3.37   **A B E** (Diabetes mellitus)
       C increased in autumn and winter
       D 10%

3.38   **C E** (Limping and joint disorder)
       A ESR usually normal
       B <5% subsequently develop features of Perthes' disease
       D X-rays typically normal

3.39   **A C E** (Meningitis and encephalitis)
       B suggestive of meningococcal disease and is not in itself a contra-indication to lumbar puncture (LP)
       D suggestive of meningitis in an infant or neonate and not a contra-indication to LP

3.40   **A E** (Muscle and neuromuscular disorders)
       B more common in girls
       C hypotonia is an uncommon presentation
       D is an autoimmune disease. There is a congenital form which is an autosomal recessive condition presenting in the newborn period, which is relatively resistant to treatment

3.41   **A C D E** (Blistering conditions)
       B if there is an associated enteropathy, a gluten-free diet is the treatment of choice; may also treat with dapsone

3.42   **B** (Abdominal pain – acute)
       A diagnosis is hardest in this age-group because abdominal signs are difficult to elicit, and previous antibiotic administration may alter the presentation
       C a low-grade fever is usual
       D a neutrophil leucocytosis is typical
       E there is no specific bleeding point

3.43 **A B C D** (Neurocutaneous syndromes)
     E   50% of children have learning difficulties

3.44 **A C D** (Eczema)
     B   erythema, vesicles, lichenification and crusting are recognized features of eczema, and may occur on the cheeks
     E   the Koebner phenomenon occurs in psoriasis, where lesions occur along the site of skin injury

3.45 **A D** (Kawasaki disease)
     B   there is no specific contra-indication to digoxin
     C   mucous membrane changes constitute a clinical criteria for diagnosis of Kawasaki disease. They are not herpetic
     E   not given routinely, the usual indications for antibiotic prophylaxis apply

3.46 **B C E** (Immunodeficiency)
     A   neutrophils have a reduced capacity to kill micro-organisms after engulfment
     D   delayed cord separation is a feature of leucocyte adhesion deficiency

3.47 **A B D E** (Liver disease)
     C   homocystinuria is not a recognized cause

3.48 **A B C D** (Congenital infection)
     E   a rash is not a specific feature

3.49 **A B C D** (Vomiting)
     E   omeprazole is a proton-pump inhibitor reducing gastric acid production. Ondansetron, a 5-HT3 inhibitor is widely used as an anti-emetic during chemotherapy

3.50 **A B D E** (HIV infection)
     C   there is a 'ground' glass appearance on X-ray

3.51 **A B C E** (Gastroenteritis)
     D   Coxsackie A16 causes hand, foot, and mouth disease

3.52 **A B D E** (Pyrexia of unknown origin)
     C   lisch nodules occur in type 1 neurofibromatosis (NF1) and are found on the iris

3.53   **A B C D** (Gastrointestinal haemorrhage)
       E   this facial rash is a feature of tuberous sclerosis

Burns J, Chapman PD, Eastham EJ. Familial adenomatous polyposis. *Archives of Disease in Childhood*, 1994; **71**: 103–7

3.54   **A D** (Jaundice)
       B   there is no evidence of haemolysis
       C   mild unconjugated hyperbilirubinaemia
       E   splenomegaly is not a feature

3.55   **C E** (Neonatal jaundice)
       A   there is a later peak and trough in the preterm infant
       B   jaundice in the first 24 hours is always pathological
       D   physiological jaundice fades by the 7th–10th day

3.56   **A B C D E** (Chronic diarrhoea)

3.57   **A B D E** (Cystic fibrosis)
       C   this is not a complication of cystic fibrosis

3.58   **B C D** (Hearing and speech)
       A   this is an 8 month milestone
       E   can be used from the age of 4 years. Methods that can be used in a neonate include auditory evoked responses

3.59   **B C E** (Antenatal diagnostics)
       A   16–18 weeks
       D   culture and analysis of amniotic cells takes 2–3 weeks

3.60   **A B E** (Headache)
       C   this is typical of headache due to raised intracranial pressure
       D   occasionally heard in the presence of an intracranial arteriovenous malformation

ANSWERS TO PAPER FOUR

The correct answers appear in bold
The topic names in brackets refer to the topics in *Key Topics in Paediatrics*

4.1 **B E** (Diabetes mellitus)
    A hypokalaemia
    C 65 ml/hour would be maintenance requirements but usually 5–10% dehydrated at presentation with DKA - need to replace deficit as well as give maintenance fluids in first 24 hours:
        maintenance = $(100 \times 10) + (50 \times 10) + (25 \times 2) = 1550$ ml/day
        + deficit (if 10% dehydrated) = 2200 ml over 24 hours
        (i.e. 156 ml/hour total)
    D no association so it is difficult to predict who is at greatest risk

4.2 **A B C D E** (Hypoglycaemia)

4.3 **A B** (Inborn errors of metabolism)
    C no particular smell, cf. maple syrup urine disease
    D not a typical feature
    E cataracts

4.4 **A B E** (Neonatal convulsions)
Haemorrhagic disease of the newborn may cause a convulsion as a result of intracranial haemorrhage
    C, D no association

4.5 **A B D E** (Calcium metabolism)
    C hyperphosphataemia

4.6 **A B C D E** (Sickle cell anaemia and thalassaemia syndromes)

4.7 **A C E** (Chronic renal failure)
    B secondary hyperparathyroidism
    D reduced calcium absorption due to low levels of 1,25 dihydroxy-vitamin D

4.8 **B E** (Neonatal respiratory distress)
    A may take 48 hours to settle
    C impossible to completely exclude infection on CXR so most are treated with antibiotics until cultures prove negative
    D delayed clearance of fetal lung fluid

4.9 **A C E** (Congenital heart disease – cyanotic)
    B right axis deviation
    D single second heart sound

4.10 A E (Polyuria and renal tubular disorders)
       B   calculi form in only 3% of affected individuals
       C   cystinosis
       D   cystinosis

4.11 A B C D E (Ataxia)

4.12 A D E (Haematuria)
       B   slowly progressive or fulminant course in some cases
       C   diffuse mesangial deposits of IgA

4.13 A B E (Anaemia)
       C   iron deficiency anaemia
       D   megaloblastic anaemia due to folate deficiency

4.14 A B (Growth – short and tall stature)
       C   initially tall compared with peers because of early pubertal growth spurt but tend not to be tall at final height due to early fusion of the epiphyses
       D   short stature
       E   usually not indicated

4.15 B C E (Thyroid disorders)
       A   anterior pituitary
       D   often worse behaviour initially

4.16 A B E (Shock)
       C   capillary refill time prolonged >2 sec
       D   oliguria usual

4.17 A B C D (Acute hemiplegia)
       E   cyanotic

4.18 B C E (Abdominal pain – recurrent)
       A   majority (>90%) non-organic or functional
       D   no difference in intelligence between affected children and controls

4.19 A B C (Asthma)
       D   suggests alternative diagnosis (e.g. cystic fibrosis)
       E   suggests structural lung disease (e.g. bronchiectasis, airway obstruction due to a foreign body)

4.20 A C E (Burns)
       B   consider if >10%, but also if smaller areas when full thickness or if site suggests poor cosmetic or functional outcome (e.g. face, hands)
       D   may be necessary if thoracic or limb burns are circumferential

4.21 **B C** (Lower respiratory tract infection)
A usually respiratory syncytial virus
D only 1–5%
E ribavirin

4.22 **A C E** (Hypertension)
B blood pressure usually normal, cf. Conn's syndrome
D hypotension

4.23 **D E** (Malignancy in childhood)
Families with Li Fraumeni syndrome (germline mutations of the p53 tumour suppressor gene) have an increased risk of cancers particularly childhood sarcomas and maternal breast cancer.
A one-third more common in boys
B ~16% of deaths – 2nd most common cause of death in this age group
C ~1200 newly diagnosed per year

4.24 **A C** (Birth injuries)
B usually unilateral, bilateral suggests a congenital defect of VIIth nerves
D damage to the lower brachial plexus roots C8,T1 results in Klumpke's palsy
E the arm affected by an Erb's palsy is held in the waiter's tip position

4.25 **A C D** (Child abuse)
B not a reliable sign as it is found in other conditions (e.g. severe constipation)
E seen 10–14 days after a fracture with callus formation from 14 days

4.26 **C D E** (Behaviour)
A occur during deep non-rapid eye movement sleep
B no recollection of sleep walking

4.27 **B D** (Chromosomal abnormalities)
A sterility is almost invariable
C 0.4 per 1000 live births
E usually normal intelligence or mild learning difficulties only

4.28 **B C E** (Demography and definitions)
A per 1000 *live* births
D number of stillbirths and deaths in the first week per 1000 *total* births

4.29 **B C** (Developmental delay and regression)
A, D, E   these are causes of global developmental delay but regression is not characteristic

4.30   **A C E** (Poisoning)
        B   all patients should be admitted and gastric lavage performed if vomiting cannot be induced
        D   phase 2 is the quiescent phase

4.31   **A B C D** (Dysmorphology and teratogenesis)
        E   not a typical feature

4.32   **B C** (Enuresis)
        A   rarely indicated
        D   desmospray is given nasally and desmotabs orally
        E   also sometimes helpful in older children

4.33   **B C E** (Failure to thrive)
        A   less than 10% have an organic cause
        D   absolute weight is not diagnostic (e.g. would be failing to thrive if weight fell from 91st to 25th centiles without ever being below 0.4th centile)

4.34   **A B C E** (Floppy infant)
        D   does not cause hypotonia

4.35   **A B E** (Hydrocephalus)
        C   restriction of upward gaze
        D   uncommon in infancy due to the ability of the skull to expand

4.36   **None true** (Immunization)
        A   suspension of killed *Bordetella pertussis* organisms
        B   combined with diphtheria and tetanus as the triple vaccine
        C   may be contra-indicated in children with evolving neurological conditions but not in Down's syndrome
        D   currently given at 2, 3 and 4 months in the UK
        E   diphtheria, tetanus and polio boosters but not pertussis

4.37   **C E** (Limping and joint disorders)
        A   most commonly large joints
        B   *Staphylococcus aureus* is the most common organism
        D   minimum 3 weeks with at least the first week being administered intravenously

4.38   **B D E** (Peripheral neuropathy)
        A   flaccid paralysis
        C   no correlation between severity and prognosis if appropriate supportive care is given

4.39 **B D** (Meningitis and encephalitis)
　　A　normal
　　C　normal or raised
　　E　low

4.40 **A B E** (Muscle and neuromuscular disorders)
　　C　difficulty in relaxing the grasp
　　D　usually associated with mild learning difficulties

4.41 **A B C D E** (Osteomyelitis)

4.42 **E** (Polyarthritis)
　　A　five or more joints affected
　　B　rarely a feature
　　C　rarely indicated
　　D　minimal systemic features, cf. Still's disease

4.43 **A C E** (Single gene defects)
　　B　autosomal recessive
　　D　X-linked dominant

4.44 **A C D E** (Upper respiratory tract infection)
　　B　surgical drainage rarely required

4.45 **A** (Constipation)
　　B　hypercalcaemia may be the cause
　　C　long courses of laxatives (1–2 years) are often needed
　　D　rectal biopsy is required
　　E　abdominal X-ray may reveal spinal anomalies and demonstrate the degree of faecal loading

4.46 **A C** (Eczema)
　　B　thrombocytopenia and eczema are features of Wiskott–Aldrich syndrome
　　D　anaemia is not a typical finding
　　E　antigliadin antibodies are found in coeliac disease and dermatitis herpetiformis

4.47 **A E** (Stridor)
　　B　the cry and cough are normal (vocal cords normal)
　　C　stridor is worse in the supine position
　　D　the infant is usually thriving

4.48   **D** (Nutrition)
- A formula milks should provide casein:whey ratios which approximate those in human milks (i.e. 40:60)
- B this is an excessive amount – volumes of 150 ml/kg/day are more appropriate
- C unmodified cow's milk should not be introduced before 1 year of age as the iron and vitamin content is too low
- E breast feeding should be promoted wherever possible – in this case the mother's anaemia should be corrected

4.49   **A C** (Developmental assessment)
- B, D would be expected at 3 years
- E   would be expected at 4 years

4.50   **A B D E** (Cleft lip and palate)
- C no association

4.51   **A C D** (Rashes and naevi)
- B the epidermal naevus syndrome is associated with developmental defects
- E these scalp lesions appear as smooth, waxy plaques – there is no haemangiomatous element

4.52   **A B D E** (Pyrexia of unknown origin)
- C pyrexia is not a feature of coelic disease

4.53   **A B C D** (Cystic fibrosis)
- E this causes respiratory illness in the immunocompromized child (e.g. HIV infection)

4.54   **A B C D E** (Gastrointestinal haemorrhage)

4.55   **A B C D E** (Jaundice)

Gregorio GV, Mieli-Vergani G. Hepatitits B infection. *Current Paediatrics*, 1995; 5: 24–7

4.56   **A B D E** (Neonatal jaundice)
- C total parenteral nutrition causes a cholestatic conjugated hyperbilirubinaemia

4.57   **A B C D** (Childhood exanthemata)
- E treatment should be with penicillin, cephalosporins or erythromycin

4.58 **A C D** (Seizures)
B typically 4–7 months
E chaotic hypsarrhythmia on EEG

4.59 **A D** (Hearing and speech)
B 7–9 months
C used to assess both expression and comprehension
E useful particularly for middle ear problems

4.60 **B C E** (Antenatal diagnostics *and* Chromosomal abnormalities)
A low AFP
D no increased risk

ANSWERS TO PAPER FIVE

The correct answers appear in bold
The topic names in brackets refer to the topics in *Key Topics in Paediatrics*

5.1 **A C D E** (Acute hemiplegia)
    B post infectious encephalitis is a recognized complication of varicella and measles but not rubella

5.2 **A B D E** (Abdominal pain – recurrent)
    C non-organic

5.3 **A C E** (Asthma)
    B nebulizers and spacer devices with face masks can be used even in neonates
    D inappropriate selection or incorrect use of inhaler device more likely

Thorax, 1993; 48: supplement S1-S24

5.4 **A C D** (Burns)
    B this is a second degree (partial thickness) burn
    E rule of nines in older children, with allowance for relatively bigger head in younger children (e.g. Lund and Browder charts)

5.5 **A C D** (Lower respiratory tract infection)
    B *Staphylococcus aureus* in infancy
    E *Pneumocystis carinii* typically affects immunocompromised patients

5.6 **B** (Children and the law)
    A followed the Warnock report, the Calman report was on higher specialist training
    C permission should be sought from the parents
    D 30 days
    E should be reviewed annually

5.7 **B E** (Haemolytic uraemic syndrome)
    A haemolytic anaemia
    C not a common feature
    D hypertension

5.8 **A B C D E** (Cerebral palsy)

5.9 C (Behaviour)
- A more common in boys
- B many are idiopathic, some are associated with other conditions (e.g. tuberous sclerosis, fragile X)
- D features usually prominent by 2–3 years of age
- E 70% have severe learning difficulties

5.10 A C D E (Birth injuries)
- B this is a 'normal' delivery

5.11 A C D (Chromosomal abnormalities)
- B typical of Edward's syndrome
- E most children with Patau's syndrome die within the first few weeks of life

5.12 D E (Congenital dislocation of the hip and talipes)
- A more common in boys
- B 50%
- C oligohydramnios

5.13 D (Demography and definitions)
- A ~one-third
- B one-quarter live in developed countries, three-quarters in developing countries
- C ~11 million
- E a GP with an average sized list (2500 patients) will have ~450 patients under 15 years

5.14 A C D E (Developmental assessment)
- B should be able to copy a cross

5.15 E (Diabetes mellitus)
- A replace deficit over 24 hours
- B insulin promotes uptake of potassium into cells
- C commence i.v. insulin at 0.1 units/kg/hour
- D bicarbonate is rarely needed

5.16 E (Enuresis)
- A 10% of children regularly wet the bed at the age of 5 years
- B more common in boys
- C only 1–2%
- D more common in lower socioeconomic groups

5.17 A B C D E (Failure to thrive)

5.18 **E** (Floppy infant)
   A autosomal recessive
   B respiratory failure
   C facial and bulbar muscles usually unaffected
   D may be profoundly floppy at birth

5.19 **B D E** (Hydrocephalus)
   A produced by the choroid plexus
   C pressure is normal

5.20 **D E** (Immunization)
   A should be given irrespective of a history of the illness
   B live attenuated MMR vaccines
   C first dose at 12–18 months

5.21 **A B D E** (Inborn errors of metabolism)
   C hypoglycaemia is a common presenting feature

5.22 **B** (Meningitis and encephalitis)
   A 10%
   C the role of steroids in reducing the inflammatory response is controversial but may be of benefit in haemophilus meningitis
   D *E. coli* and other Gram negative organisms, group B streptococcus and *Listeria monocytogenes* are the most common aetiological agents in the neonatal period
   E cefotaxime is currently the drug of choice

5.23 **E** (Muscle and neuromuscular disorders)
   A at least 60%
   B falls
   C usually presents in the first 5 years of life
   D sex-linked recessive

5.24 **B C D E** (Osteomyelitis)
   A the most common is *Staphylococcus aureus*

5.25 **A C E** (Poisoning)
   B, D are not contra-indications

5.26 **A B D** (Polyarthritis)
   C usually no systemic symptoms
   E usually 1–5 years

5.27 **B E** (Single gene defects)
- A sex-linked dominant
- C sex-linked recessive
- D autosomal dominant

5.28 **B E** (Sudden infant death syndrome)
- A prone sleeping is a risk factor, supine sleeping is advised
- C young maternal age
- D there is a lack of evidence for the protective effect of breast feeding

5.29 **A D E** (Upper respiratory tract infection)
- B ~ 4 upper respiratory tract infections per year
- C usually viral

5.30 **C D E** (Vision)
- A usually concomitant
- B 3–5%

5.31 **B C D E** (Immunodeficiency)
- A tonsils are usually absent

5.32 **A B C D E** (Congenital infection)

5.33 **A B D E** (HIV infection)
- C polycythaemia is not a recognized feature

5.34 **A B D** (Gastroenteritis)
- C Sigmoid volvulus typically occurs in the elderly. A chronically loaded colon, such as in constipation, would predispose to volvulus
- E other viruses are implicated (e.g. varicella, Coxsackie)

5.35 **B C D E** (Nutrition)
- A the hindmilk has a higher fat content

5.36 **A B D E** (Congenital heart disease – cyanotic)
- C polycythaemia is usual

5.37 **A C** (Growth – short and tall stature)
- B normal velocity for pubertal stage
- D good height prognosis
- E usually slim build, cf. endocrine causes of short stature

5.38 **A B C D E** (Malignancy in childhood)

5.39 **A B C E** (Cardiopulmonary resuscitation)
VF may complicate near-drowning due to hypothermia
D adrenaline given if unresponsive to 2 J/kg twice followed by 4 J/kg once

5.40 **A E** (Sickle cell anaemia and thalassaemia syndromes)
B raised HbF 15–100%, normally <5%
C usually presents in the first year of life
D more common in Mediterranean and Asian races, cf. sickle cell disease

5.41 **B** (Limping and joint disorders)
A 10–15 years
C associated with gonadal immaturity
D pain in hip, thigh or knee with no swelling
E 20%

5.42 **B D E** (Calcium metabolism)
Some primitive renal tumours secrete a PTH-related protein which causes hypercalcaemia
A rare in childhood
C suppresses PTH secretion

5.43 **A E** (Purpura and bruising)
B <1%
C not essential in all cases but, if considering steroid treatment, bone marrow must be examined first to exclude leukaemia
D normal or increased megakaryocyte numbers

5.44 **C E** (Solid tumours)
A most affected children are <5 years old
B rare presenting feature – usually just asymptomatic abdominal mass
D aniridia

5.45 **A C** (Congenital heart disease – acyanotic)
B murmur arises from increased flow across the pulmonary valve
D uncommon, usually requires surgery
E full immunization should be encouraged

5.46 **A B C E** (Childhood exanthemata)
D measles has an incubation period of 10 days

5.47 **A B C E** (Gastrointestinal haemorrhage *and* Abdominal pain – acute)
D there are no cutaneous stigmata of Meckel's diverticulum. Peri-oral pigmentation occurs in Peutz–Jeger syndrome, which is associated with small bowel polyps

5.48   **A D E** (Jaundice)
       B   there is no vertical transmission
       C   there is no carrier state

5.49   **B C E** (Neonatal jaundice)
       A   biliary atresia is an inflammatory obstruction of the extrahepatic bile ducts, and is not an inherited disease
       D   the infants look normal – see reference

Howard ER. Surgery for biliary atresia. *Current Paediatrics*, 1995; **5**: 28–31

5.50   **A C D E** (Pyrexia of unknown origin)
       B   not a recognized complication

5.51   **D** (Rashes and naevi)
       A   they occasionally occur in Caucasian races
       B   they fade by the end of the first decade
       C   there is no associated spinal lesion
       E   melanocytic naevi (moles), and the giant pigmented naevi in particular, may undergo malignant change

5.52   **A B D E** (Ataxia)
       C   hypertension may cause vomiting, visual disturbance and seizures

5.53   **B C D** (Neurocutaneous syndromes)
       A   inheritance is X-linked dominant, usually lethal in males
       E   polycystic kidneys are a feature of tuberous sclerosis, in which there is renal involvement in 80% of cases

5.54   **A B C E** (Chronic diarrhoea)
       D   *Helicobacter pylori* causes chronic gastritis and peptic ulcer disease

5.55   **A B C D** (Cystic fibrosis)
       E   nasal polyps are found in cystic fibrosis

5.56   **A B C D E** (Seizures)
       Breath holding may cause a reflex anoxic seizure

5.57   **A C E** (Constipation)
       B   early withdrawal of laxatives frequently leads to relapse – may need to be continued for a year or more
       D   stool softener

5.58   **B C E** (Hearing and speech)
       A   deafness is associated with glomerulonephritis in Alport's syndrome
       D   detected only in the first 6 months of life

5.59 **A C D E** (Developmental delay and regression)
B average age of independent walking is 15 months, developmental delay suggested if not walking by 18 months

5.60 **A B D E** (Hypoglycaemia)
Septo-optic dysplasia (the anatomical triad of optic nerve hypoplasia, absence of the septum pellucidum and agenesis or thinning of the corpus callosum) is associated with hypothalamic-pituitary dysfunction. Deliberate administration of insulin to a child who is not diabetic is a recognized form of Munchausen by proxy
C Reye's syndrome not Rett's syndrome

ANSWERS TO PAPER SIX

The topic names in brackets refer to the topics in *Key Topics in Paediatrics*

6.1 (Adrenal disorders)
   A Congenital adrenal hyperplasia – most commonly due to 21 hydroxylase deficiency
   B Plasma 17 hydroxyprogesterone level – will be raised. The specific enzyme defect can be confirmed by urinary steroid profile
   C Rehydration and correction of hypoglycaemia/hyponatraemia with saline and dextrose. Steroid replacement with a glucocorticoid (hydrocortisone) and a mineralocorticoid (fludrocortisone) +/- sodium supplements

6.2 (Purpura and bruising *and* Leukaemia and lymphoma)
   A The two most common causes of thrombocytopenia in childhood are ITP and acute leukaemia. The presence of neutropenia makes leukaemia the most likely diagnosis
   B Bone marrow aspiration to confirm the diagnosis, lumbar puncture to look for leukaemic blasts in the CSF (CNS disease at diagnosis is a poor prognostic indicator), CXR to look for mediastinal widening (suggests T-cell ALL)

6.3 (Growth – short and tall stature)
   A Parental heights to predict adult height potential, previous height measurements for growth velocity calculation
   B Thyroid function tests (hypothyroidism), karyotype (Turner's syndrome), bone age (constitutional delay in growth and puberty)
   C Coarctation of the aorta causes hypertension in the upper limbs and is found in 10% of girls with Turner's syndrome. Marked anxiety as the cause is excluded by the fact that she remains hypertensive on repeated measurements. Chronic renal failure, which is a cause of growth failure and hypertension is excluded by the normal renal function tests

6.4 (Diabetes mellitus)
   A Diabetic ketoacidosis
   B (1) Airway – is the child maintaining his airway? (2) Breathing – is his respiratory effort adequate to maintain his oxygenation? (3) Circulation – is he shocked (pulse, blood pressure, capillary return, assessment of the degree of dehydration)? (4) Conscious level
   C Commence rehydration with normal saline then start an insulin infusion
   D Cerebral oedema, hypokalaemia

6.5 (Abdominal pain - Acute)
   A Rectal examination might reveal a bloody stool ('redcurrant jelly' stool) suggestive of an intussusception
   B Acceptable answers include plain abdominal X-ray (?abdominal US), urinalysis, urea and electrolytes
   C This picture would be typical of an intussusception
   D Rehydrate the child then proceed to barium or air enema to confirm the diagnosis. Hydrostatic reduction may be attempted as the history is relatively short and the child is not shocked. Surgical reduction would be indicated if this fails

6.6 (Thyroid disorders)
   A The child is only taking her medication intermittently. Difficulty getting a child to take medications at this age is common but the importance of compliance for her growth and development must be emphasized to her parents

6.7 (Congenital heart disease – cyanotic)
   A Transposition of the great arteries (TGA) with a ventricular septal defect (VSD). Profound cyanosis in the absence of respiratory distress makes a diagnosis of cyanotic congenital heart disease very likely and TGA would be the most likely defect before the ECG result is known. If there was no associated VSD the baby would have collapsed acutely as the ductus arteriosus closed
   B Single second heart sound, pansystolic murmur loudest at the left sternal edge
   C +340° is a superior axis due to extreme left axis deviation. This ECG is typical of tricuspid atresia
   D Commence a prostaglandin E2 infusion to re-open the ductus arteriosus

6.8 (Haemolytic uraemic syndrome)
   A Haemolytic uraemic syndrome
   B Full blood count will show thrombocytopenia and a microangiopathic haemolytic anaemia. Urea and electrolytes will confirm a degree of renal failure. Verotoxin-producing *E.coli* might be isolated from the stools
   C This is likely to be a flow murmur secondary to anaemia

6.9 (Puberty – precocious and delayed)

A Acceptable answers include blood pressure measurement, examination of the genitalia for cliteromegaly, calculation of growth velocity, palpation for an abdominal mass
The differential diagnosis is between simple premature adrenarche and an abnormal source of androgens (e.g. congenital adrenal hyperplasia, adrenal tumour). Hypertension, accelerated growth velocity, cliteromegaly, or an abdominal mass would point towards the latter

B Investigations might include plasma androgens (e.g. DHEAS, androstenedione, testosterone), 17-hydroxyprogesterone, urinary steroid profile, bone age, abdominal ultrasound

6.10 (Nephrotic syndrome)

A A mixed picture of nephrotic syndrome with nephritic features (hypertension, microscopic haematuria, degree of renal failure)

B Hypovolaemia or peritonitis

C It suggests that the child's kidneys are maximally retaining salt and water in an attempt to compensate for critical hypovolaemia

6.11 (Kawasaki disease)

A Kawasaki disease

B There is no specific test – the diagnostic criteria are clinical features and exclusion of other conditions such as staphlococcal or streptococcal infection, measles, and drug reactions. Fbc may show a raised platelet count

C High dose intravenous immunoglobulin and high dose oral aspirin

D Cardiovascular complications including coronary artery aneurysms, myocarditis and pericarditis occur in 20–30% of cases. The mortality is 1–2% due to coronary complications. Early diagnosis and treatment (within the first 10 days of the illness) may reduce the incidence of cardiac complications

6.12 (Neonatal jaundice)

A Conjugated/unconjugated serum bilirubin. With bilirubin in the urine it is likely that >80% of the total serum bilirubin will be conjugated

B The baby is at risk of hypoglycaemia and bleeding due to liver dysfunction

C The main differential diagnosis is between biliary atresia (extrahepatic cholestasis) and intrahepatic cholestasis due to various conditions (e.g. galactosaemia, congenital hypothyroidism, congenital infection)

6.13 (Calcium metabolism *and* Single gene defects)
- **A** X-linked hypophosphataemic (vitamin D resistant) rickets – in this condition rickets is due to defective re-absorption of phosphate from the proximal renal tubules. The child has disproportionate short stature with a normal sitting height but short standing height due to bowing of his legs. Typically this bowing develops as the child starts to weight bear on his legs
- **B** It is an X-linked dominant condition. Affected males have only affected daughters, whereas there is a 50% risk of a child of either sex inheriting the condition from an affected female. In this case the mother is extremely short so it seems likely that she is the affected parent. There is therefore a 50% chance of the younger sister being affected

6.14 (Arrhythmias)
- **A** Congenital complete heart block
- **B** Anti-Ro and anti-DNA antibodies. Congenital complete heart block occurs in babies of mothers who have a connective tissue disorder (especially systemic lupus erythematosis), probably secondary to the passive transfer of anti-Ro or anti-DNA antibodies across the placenta

6.15 (no specific topic)
- **A** Respiratory alkalosis
- **B** Hyperventilation probably due to hysterical overbreathing

6.16 (Developmental assessment *and* Developmental delay and regression)
- **A** The child is showing gross motor delay. Her fine motor skills and language development are appropriate for a developmental age of 22 months, whereas creeping on hands and knees is found at a developmental age of 11 months

6.17 (Haemophilia and Christmas disease)
- **A** Haemophilia A or Christmas disease
- **B** Measurement of factor VIII and factor IX levels

6.18 (Single gene defects *and* Chromosomal abnormalities)
- **A** X-linked recessive
- **B** Fragile X syndrome

6.19 (Anaemia)
  A Blackfan–Diamond syndrome (congenital hypoplastic anaemia) – in this syndrome the red cell aplasia usually presents during infancy. It is associated with other congenital abnormalities in 25% of cases, including skeletal abnormalities, cleft lip and palate, neck webbing, cardiac defects, hypocalcaemia, and hypogammaglobulinaemia. Chromosomal abnormalities may also be found

Alter, BP. The bone marrow failure syndromes. In: Nathan DG and Oski FA (eds) *Haematology in Infancy and Childhood.* Philadelphia: Saunders, 1987; 197–206.

6.20 (Inborn errors of metabolism *and* Neonatal jaundice)
  A Clinitest® detects reducing sugars and Clinistix® is specific for glucose. Galactose in the urine will give a positive Clinitest result
  B Galactosaemia
  C A strict lactose and galactose free diet is required. Untreated galactosaemia leads to severe learning difficulties, behaviour problems, and liver cirrhosis

6.21 (Calcium metabolism)
  A William's syndrome – idiopathic hypercalcaemia of infancy, characteristic elfin facies, moderate learning difficulties and cardiac defects
  B Supravalvular aortic stenosis is the most common heart defect associated with this syndrome

6.22 (Congenital heart disease – cyanotic)
  A Tetralogy of Fallot – there is a step down in saturation at the level of the left ventricle suggesting a right-to-left shunt at ventricular level. The right ventricular pressure is elevated but the pulmonary artery pressure is not, suggesting the presence of pulmonary stenosis

6.23 (Chromosomal abnormalities *and* Antenatal diagnostics)
  A The mother has a balanced translocation involving chromosomes 14 and 21. She has only 45 chromosomes as she has one chromosome 21, one chromosome 14 and one fused chromosome 14,21 but there is no significant loss of chromosomal material
  B The risk of a having another child with an unbalanced trisomy 21 in any future pregnancy is 10–15%, so amniocentesis or chorionic villous biopsy should be offered
6.24 (Neonatal respiratory distress)

    A Mixed respiratory and metabolic acidosis with moderate hypoxia
    B (1) Blockage or displacement of the endotracheal tube – check position and patency and if in any doubt replace it.
(2) Pneumothorax – if detected by cold light transillumination or confirmed by CXR insert a chest drain.
In both situations it may be necessary to increase the ventilation by increasing the peak inspiratory pressure (e.g. to 24–26 mmHg). The metabolic acidosis might be reduced by giving colloid to improve the peripheral perfusion

6.25 (Coeliac disease *and* Failure to thrive)
    A Coeliac disease – she has iron deficiency anaemia and a degree of hypoalbuminaemia suggesting malabsorption. Together with the clinical picture these would be typical of coeliac disease
    B Antigliadin, antiendomysium and antireticulin antibodies can be measured as a screening test but the definitive diagnostic test is a jejunal biopsy
    C Gluten-free diet, iron supplementation